THANK YOU!

Thank you for reading this short book on hormone optimization for women. As a special thank you for spending your precious time with me, I'd like to offer you some free gifts.

Please head over to:

https://PEMABioIdentical.com/book

for additional resources and materials to help you on your journey.

CLIENT TESTIMONIALS

"For over 10 years now, I have dabbled with hormone replacement therapy to address my extremely low levels as I transitioned through perimenopause, combined with high levels of stress in my life. Crippling fatigue, anxiety and depression, migraines, lack of vigor, and overall symptoms of poor aging were crushing me mentally and physically.

"Utilizing low levels of BHRT helped a little with some symptoms but did not reach the therapeutic levels I needed to feel, look and perform at my best. And oftentimes, the side effects caused me to stop therapy without further discussion of proper dosing and delivery. Now on appropriate doses of testosterone, estradiol and progesterone for my personal needs, I am finally feeling like myself again. Adding on thyroid supplementation despite other providers insisting my levels were "normal" has been a game changer. The approach to using BHRT as a means of increasing my healthspan, under the care of a team that understands proper dosing and necessary testing to address different phases of life, has given me back vitality, strength, endurance, and the confidence to age gracefully."

—Julie Wallace

"I'm so glad to be on bioidentical hormones for bone strengthening and the bonus of having sexual desire and an active sex life again, which is very nice for a postmenopausal woman in my mid-60's. Thanks for that—it was a bonus!"

—Pat York

"I recently took a photo of myself in a bathing suit on a family trip to Punta Cana. It's the only time in my life I didn't have to go on a "diet" before vacation. At 52-years-old, I'm eating more than I ever have, but I'm eating good, nourishing foods. I have stopped "babying" my spine and started lifting heavier and more often. My sleep has changed DRAMATICALLY for the better since getting on accurate dosages of estradiol, testosterone and progesterone. My gut health has also improved significantly - so much so that I can't believe I used to live the way I was living. I am diligent about taking the recommended supplements, and though my life can be (admittedly) quite stressful, I'm always working on ways to decrease anxiety. I have learned an inordinate, life-changing amount since signing on with OHH. My osteoporosis diagnosis was a wakeup call, and I'm beyond grateful to Dr. Doug and his AMAZING team as they help me respond to the call."

—Robyn Coden

"Dr. Doug, I would love to share my journey so far with your program! It truly has been life changing! It was definitely the best decision I made to take action on my bone health journey! I went from feeling discouraged by only option offered was drugs, and being told that lifestyle doesn't have that much impact. To now being a part of your program, learning that there is SO much that I can do to support my bones! I appreciate the thoughtfulness in the design of your program to support all the many areas that impact bones and overall health! Working on gut health and detox this last month with Kerri, and sleep with Julia has been more pieces of the puzzle of areas that I didn't realize I needed so much work in.

"Every day when I login to chronometer and see the banner 'A Patient of OHH', I am so very grateful to be a part of your program and reminds me to show up again every day to put the work in to support my health and my bones. I had very little knowledge of the menopause HRT world before starting. Which was good in that I didn't have any expectations, except bone support. I am still amazed at the difference in anxiety, overall brain function, and just feeling more like myself on HRT. Truly a game changer! I am glad that you don't recommend only taking for a certain time. You got me hooked, definitely don't want to give up my hormones! I appreciate so much my first experience with HRT was with a provider that really knows how to dose and manage. Talking to friends that didn't have such a great experience with HRT. I feel so blessed to get such a great provider that does so much research and manages so thoughtfully! I am so grateful to have such a robust plan and incredible support to be able to turn around my bone health and overall health! And other areas like my blood sugars have gotten so much better! I will definitely write the review, it just maybe a bit long! Forever grateful."

—Beth Zimbicki

"HRT has been life changing for me. I feel more vibrant, more lean, more energy and just overall vitality and life coming back to me."

—Cindy M.

ALSO BY DR. DOUG:

*The Osteoporosis Breakthrough:
The Natural Way to Reverse Causes of
Bone Loss and Build Strong Bones!*

Hormone Replacement for Women Is Outdated

TOP 10 REASONS WHY YOUR HORMONES ARE FAILING YOU

An Outsider's Guide to What's Wrong With Women's Hormone Prescribing Today!

Dr. Doug Lucas

PUBLISHED BY DR. DOUG LUCAS

Copyright © 2024

Printed in the United States of America

All rights reserved. Without limiting the rights under copyright reserved above, no part of this book may be reproduced, stored or introduced into a retrieval system, or transmitted, in any form or by any means (electronic, mechanical, photocopying, recording or otherwise), without the prior written permission of both the copyright owner and the publisher.

082024

DISCLAIMER:

The contents of this book are for general informational purposes only. Please consult with your healthcare team before implementing any tools discussed in this book. No doctor-patient relationship (DPR) can be formed by reading this text, and no specific recommendations are being made. The reading of this book is not designed to constitute medical care and should not substitute for medical care.

CONTENTS

Part 1—Welcome

Foreword by Maria Claps and Kristin Johnson 1

Foreword by Dr. Salomé Masghati.............................5

Who Should Read This Book? 9

My Promise to You 13

Part 2—Top 10 Reasons Your Hormones Are Failing You

Reason #1–Patriarchy, Misogyny and Confusion ..19

Reason #2–Not Using Estrogen Due to Fear of Breast Cancer and Blood Clots 31

Reason #3–Not Using Progesterone Because You Don't Have a Uterus 45

Reason #4–Ignoring Stress and Adrenal Health.....53

Reason #5–Ignoring Testosterone...........................59

Reason #6–You're "Too Old" to Start HRT or "Too Old" to Continue HRT 87

Reason #7–Maybe You Simply Need More? 99

Reason #8–Maybe You Need to Menstruate? 105

Reason #9–You're Struggling to Put It All Together! 117

Reason #10–You Don't Have Access! 127

Part 3—The Path Forward

Introducing PEMA BioIdentical 135

Who Is Dr. Doug? 137

Resources..141

References 145

ACKNOWLEDGMENTS

First and foremost, I MUST acknowledge my children and wife who tolerated the late nights, weekend hours and multitude of conversations around the topic of hormone replacement I've had at the dinner table. I am grateful for their tolerance, humor and patience as I take time from them to give to you.

My remarkable team of PAs, NPs, RDs, coaches and patient-care advocates that allow me to practice in the way that I believe people should be cared for. This team of compassionate women mirrors the need for the content in this book both with the patients they serve and in many of their own lives.

My longtime friends and leadership team members at both Optimal Human Health and PEMA BioIdentical, Teresa Bowser and Breta Alstrom, who share their remarkable talents for development and organization. These two women have helped me lead from the start and have shaped the foundation of the platforms we build on today.

My patients, HealthSpan Nation members, Instagram followers and YouTube subscribers. All of you are a strong impetus behind this creation. We read thousands of your YouTube comments and Instagram DMs describing the difficulties you have getting the care you need. Your requests and demands for a better way have pushed us to create a solution to serve you better. We have to do better. I hope you can find what you are looking for here.

DEDICATION

I dedicate this book to my wife, partner and best friend, Dr. Ashley Lucas. Her support, trust and belief in my mission provide the foundation of my professional journey. As I was her test patient for her company, PHD Weight Loss and Nutrition, she is becoming mine. Her challenges and fears mirror the challenges of the patients we serve at PEMA BioIdentical. Her experience and those of my patients are painted all over the intensity in which I pursue the truth around hormone optimization and replacement.

PART 1

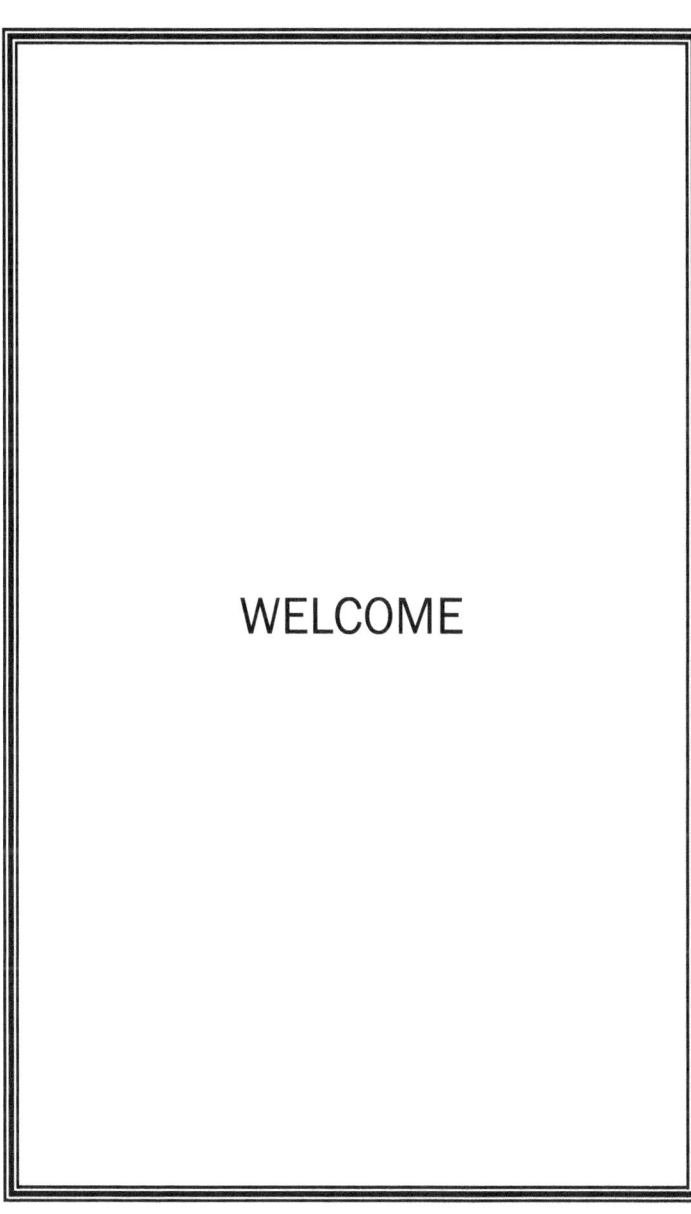

FOREWORD BY
MARIA CLAPS, FDN-P
KRISTIN JOHNSON, FNTP, JD

We first "met" Dr. Doug in the online space when his Instagram account came to our attention as a doctor who stood out from the menopause pack due to his willingness to think bigger than the oft-circulated yet little-pondered "acceptable" talking points on critical women's health topics.

The moment we became instant friends was when we asked him his thoughts on compounded hormones and he said he was a fan because "commercial products usually don't provide women with enough benefits." Stop the presses! Not only did he recognize the "benefit" of hormone therapy, but also the word "symptom" was not a part of our conversation. Had we asked this question to any number of popular menopause doctor accounts, we'd likely have received a canned response along the lines of "the guidelines say...." Yawn. This is exactly what we mean when we say that Dr. Lucas is willing to think outside the "acceptable" talking points promulgated by doctors who don't dare stray, even a little bit, from medical society guidelines. As you will soon have the benefit of reading via this thoughtful and compact book, Dr. Lucas is a critical thinker who incorporates the most up-to-date research in his recommendations but is not constrained by such guidelines when they don't inherently make sense or provide the best outcome for women's long-term health and vitality.

Dr. Doug Lucas brings exceptional expertise to this book on hormone replacement therapy for women. As a retired orthopedic surgeon, he has dedicated decades to mastering the complexities of the human body. His founding of Optimal Human Health reflects his commitment to a holistic approach, targeting the root causes of health issues, including hormonal decline in midlife. Through his YouTube channel, HealthSpan Nation, Dr. Lucas shares his extensive knowledge and practical advice, empowering a wider audience to achieve optimal health and longevity. His distinguished medical background and passion for preventive care uniquely qualify him to guide readers on their journey to better hormonal health and overall well-being.

Like us, and unlike the "must-not-stray-from-medical-society-guidelines-whatsoever" doctors who claim to be all about women's health yet have no problem offering the birth control pill to a woman in her 50s (when what she really needs is real hormones), we are passionate about a better healthspan for midlife women, something different than longevity. Longevity simply refers to the length of life, or lifespan, but healthspan refers to how long you will be able to stay healthy during your lifespan. For this reason, we were thrilled when Dr. Lucas asked us for our thoughts on physiologic rhythmic dosing of hormones. During the development of this book, we had the privilege of sharing insights and experiences with Dr. Lucas on the physiologic replacement of hormones based on our own personal HRT experiences as well as our work with thousands of women we've been able to guide through this process and the clinical experience of the mentors from whom we've been blessed to learn from. Our conversations have been instrumental in shaping some of the concepts presented here.

It's been an enriching experience to contribute to Dr. Lucas's exploration and presentation of hormone replacement therapy for women that goes beyond the standard, static dosed HRT. We are confident that his dedication and the collaborative efforts reflected in this book will provide readers with invaluable guidance on their journey to optimal health and open their eyes to the many options that they have. If you want to have a deeper understanding of standard issue hormone therapy and its many limitations, you're going to love this book. Happy learning!

—Maria Claps, FDN-P
—Kristin Johnson, FNTP, JD

FOREWORD BY SALOMÉ MASGHATI, MD

In the realm of bone health and wellness, few voices are as authoritative and insightful as Dr. Doug Lucas. Through his pioneering work in osteoporosis management for midlife women, he has not only built an empire but has fundamentally reshaped our understanding of how hormones impact bone health and beyond.

As a gynecologist and surgeon deeply invested in disease prevention and health optimization, I recognize the profound significance of hormone balance in women's health. Dr. Lucas shares this understanding, and in his latest work, he masterfully navigates the complex landscape of hormones with precision and clarity.

This book is a beacon of knowledge, where landmark studies are dissected, myths are dispelled, and the pivotal role of hormones in every facet of our body's function is illuminated. Dr. Lucas is renowned for his straightforward approach, distilling decades of research into practical insights that resonate with both medical professionals and individuals navigating their own health journey.

The heart of this book delves into the physiologic levels of estradiol and cycling progesterone—topics that spark controversy but are crucial to understand. Dr. Lucas brings these subjects to light with clarity and simplicity, making the complex world of hormones accessible to everyone.

Both Dr. Lucas and I began our careers as surgeons, trained to believe that healing meant using your surgical knife. Today, we share a belief that true healing lies in disease prevention and health optimization. This shift in perspective has fueled our passion for empowering others with the knowledge to take charge of their health. Together, we are exploring the world of rhythmic and physiologic hormones and are on a similar journey to uncover the best ways to support overall well-being for women.

Whether you are a healthcare provider seeking deeper insights or someone exploring ways to optimize health through hormone balance, this book will undoubtedly become an indispensable resource. It is with great pleasure and confidence that I commend Dr. Doug Lucas new book for his expertise, his dedication to women's health, and his invaluable contribution to our understanding of hormones.

—Salomé Masghati, MD
Gynecologist and Surgeon

WHO SHOULD READ THIS BOOK?

This short book was written for women who are considering hormone replacement or are already on hormone replacement but don't feel as good as they think they should. Over the last two decades, we have seen a FAILURE of the medical system to recognize and adequately treat many of the symptoms of the hormone changes that accompany menopause. Common hormone therapy may address the symptoms of night sweats, hot flashes and vaginal dryness, which can be debilitating, but other disturbingly common symptoms of reduced energy, brain fog, poor sleep, body composition changes, loss of muscle mass, reduced or absent libido, reduced sexual satisfaction and more are rarely discussed by most providers that prescribe hormones.

The vast majority of medical doctors, regardless of specialty, are not adequately trained in up-to-date research on hormone optimization and replacement. The research over the last 20 years can not only address the causes of symptoms of hormone imbalance but also provides data on the benefits of hormones for heart and brain health. My patients, YouTube subscribers and HealthSpan Nation members all consistently report that they feel like they have experienced gaslighting, dismissal and downright denial of care when trying to address symptoms and health goals with their doctors. Many report that their doctors would rather prescribe an antidepressant than consider hormone optimization or replacement. They refuse to order blood tests and explore the possibility that their prescribed treatment isn't meeting their patient's needs. These same women also report that they feel left on their own to explore the possible options outside of the traditional medical system, which leaves them feeling overwhelmed due to the numerous and often conflicting messages they receive. They often end up frustrated and stop pursuing the care they think they need, or even worse, submit to a therapy that ends up being harmful or causing unnecessary side effects.

Women come to me with so many questions about the potential risks and different options of replacement or optimization. With commercial and bioidentical options, over-the-counter creams, pellets and supplements all marketed to consumers, it's no wonder they feel confused, scared and unsure of where to turn. If this is you or someone you care about, this book will help to clarify the confusion and hopefully demonstrate a path forward to potentially relieve the fatigue, brain fog, loss of vitality or whichever symptoms bother you most. I urge you to spend the little precious time you have to educate yourself on the REAL risks and benefits based on up-to-date literature of hormone replacement. This last year, we have seen several landmark studies that you must hear about when making decisions around when to start hormone therapy and what options to consider.

MY PROMISE TO YOU

I admit openly that I am an unlikely advocate for women's health and hormone therapy. I'm an orthopedic surgeon and a man in his mid-40s. I won't personally go through menopause or suffer from the deficits in women's medical care that is so rampant in our country and even worse elsewhere in the world.

However, as a champion for comprehensive osteoporosis management, a board-certified and fellowship-trained functional-medicine physician, and husband to an amazing woman experiencing some of these symptoms herself as well as a father to a little girl who will face the unknown challenges of a new generation, I find myself compelled and called to write this book.

Early in training, I was fearful of stepping into the controversial arena of hormone replacement conversations. It seemed off limits to me and an area that should only be debated by doctors in the OBGYN and endocrinology specialties, as if somehow I didn't have the ability to understand the research or treatment options despite a decade on the research committee of an orthopedic society and publishing over a dozen of my own peer-reviewed articles and book chapters. I tentatively entered the hormone discussion out of necessity for my osteoporosis patients. They were often unable to find a suitable care provider and desperately needed the support.

As is true with everything in my life, I didn't just dabble in the space, I jumped in with both feet and consumed research, went through a fellowship and received a board certification so that I could feel confident in my recommendations and truly understand the issues and risks around hormones for women. As I cautiously throw my hat in the ring, I realize that many of the new popular female thought leaders that I found so intimidating are quoting data and guidelines from 20 years ago and fail to see how they themselves are propagating the same message from the patriarchy they state they oppose. I find the messaging disturbing, inaccurate and sad.

My promise to you is that I will bring my experience as a researcher, critic, author, husband, father and advocate for women's health to this book. I have sculpted an approach to hormone therapy that focuses on customized options and biomarker-driven dosing using updated research and my team's shared clinical experience.

I also promise to be openly critical of those organizations and industries that continue to oppress women's health through guidelines and recommendations that don't line up with the available and current literature. We are building a community of enlightened patients, members and followers. I once felt that as an outsider, I had no place talking about women's hormones, and I'm sure I'll receive some feedback offering that confirmation. But I realize that it will take an outsider to have the unbiased views required to wave through the mess that is the field of hormone therapy.

If you are considering hormone replacement or are not feeling as good as you think you should on hormone replacement, I strongly urge you to read this book and join me in my mission to educate women and help them to optimize their health through appropriate discussions of the options, risks and benefits of optimal hormone therapy. We need you feeling your best, and poor prescribing from your doctor shouldn't slow you down. We are going to review the top 10 reasons why your hormone replacement (or lack thereof) is failing you. Let's go.

PART 2

TOP 10 REASONS YOUR HORMONES ARE FAILING YOU

REASON #1

PATRIARCHY, MISOGYNY AND CONFUSION

We are all aging. If we are fortunate enough to walk the earth another day, we cannot avoid the impact of time. Despite all the advances, the media hype and social media claims, no one is turning back the clock on aging. Not really or at least not yet. Each season of life brings about a unique set of circumstances that we get to learn about and handle in our own unique way. Some seasons are harder than others, and some transitions are more difficult. For women, the midlife and beyond can represent an especially challenging and significant period of transition, physically, emotionally and often spiritually. It is a time when hormonal changes can have a profound impact on a woman's well-being, yet it is also a phase of life that has often been marginalized and misunderstood within the broader landscape of healthcare in the United States and worldwide.

As a physician specializing in health optimization and driven by a passion for educating and engaging with a wider audience, my mission is to shed light on topics that have long been shrouded in misconception, fear and confusion. Through the fruit of the extensive research my team and I have done for our YouTube channels and podcasts, I have witnessed the power of knowledge and the tremendous impact of empowering individuals to take control of their health and well-being. Our patients, members, subscribers and followers are empowered to take control of their lives and optimize their hormones through the lens of living better, longer. Living as well as we can for as long as we can is the defining characteristic of healthspan and the foundation of my mission to research and educate. This book is an extension of that mission, aimed at arming women with the information they need to make informed decisions about their hormonal health.

As we begin to dig into the top reasons your hormone replacement may be failing you, let's first discuss some of the root causes of all the confusion. Why is it so hard to talk about hormones? There are SO MANY issues to discuss, but in my opinion, the root cause of this issue goes way back in time. Patriarchal societies are notorious for misogyny, and this has been going on for centuries. Similarly, in medicine, the marginalization of women has persisted from the beginning of patient care. Even in modern medicine, research and treatment have been biased towards men, with women's unique physiology and health needs overlooked, or at a minimum, underrepresented. Women are often treated as small men, which clearly is a gross error in patient care. This bias toward men in research and development has had far-reaching consequences, leaving women grappling with unanswered questions, misdiagnoses, and suboptimal care. It is imperative that we address this disparity head-on now and advocate for a more inclusive and equitable approach to women's health. Women are not small men, and we shouldn't treat them as such.

Throughout the pages of this book, we will delve into the intricacies of hormone optimization and replacement, exploring the science behind it, the potential benefits, and the considerations that every woman should be aware of. At the beginning of midlife (which we define as around 40 years old), most women are still cycling regularly. However, it is around this time that natural shifts in hormone balance frequently occur. Statistically, women go through menopause around 51 years of age, as defined by the point at which 12 months pass without a menstrual cycle. While this definition seems clear-cut, the reality is that women may go through hormonal changes for a decade or more before this final definition rings true for them. During this season, they may experience "perimenopause" symptoms of anxiety, depression, weight gain, body-composition changes, fatigue, lethargy and sexual dysfunction, which are often dismissed or treated with pharmaceuticals, like antidepressants or antianxiety drugs. Hormone dysfunction is rarely considered or even tested for in women with these complaints. They are left to suffer in silence. What's so insidious about this "treatment" is that the vast majority of doctors don't even know they are doing something that may be harming their patients. Their training and the established medical model teaches oppression of women to clinical providers, and they pass this along to their patients without an understanding of what the root cause of the problem is and without the knowledge or tools to treat it if they did!

To make matters worse, the experiences of perimenopause and menopause seem to be more challenging than ever before. Some would argue that we are simply hearing more open discussion of the problem, which is true, and it's about time. But I see this as a sign of a larger problem. I'm married to a woman in this season of her life, and I see her struggles mirrored in my patients every day. Perimenopause, in particular, has become more challenging than ever before because It's during this time in our modern society that women are often put into a difficult social position. Women in our culture in their 30's, 40's and 50's are often dealing with the stresses of kids, careers, spouses, parents and more. Women take on tremendous and often unrealistic roles in modern families, and around midlife, it starts to show. Kids may still be young and rely heavily on their mom, especially in households where the traditional masculine and feminine roles put the stress from this role primarily on women. Even in these traditional households, women often are not only working outside the home to help make ends meet financially but are also often pursuing demanding careers.

I'm all for equality and support women's rights in the workplace, but adding a demanding career on top of the patriarchal archetypal household division of labor creates an imbalance that will likely result in negative health consequences for the women involved. This can be a challenging conversation for men in my generation who were raised with clear expectations of marriage. Many times, I hear the story of women continuing to shoulder the burden of childcare and maintaining the home despite having a career that is every bit as challenging as her spouse or oftentimes more so. This same season of life may also present the need to take care of aging parents, another role that is often shouldered by women. All of these responsibilities can stack up quickly and in a way that many women feel they can't change. We will explore how these stressors impact women's hormones in future chapters. It will be eye-opening!

Fortunately, there are tools unique to women that can not only help you to survive these times but also ultimately thrive! Please hear me as I go through this. I am in NO WAY saying that women are weaker than men. I'm saying that women are different from men. Stress impacts female sex hormones differently than it does men's. I like to consider myself enlightened to the superior nature of women in a partnership. I consider myself the king of my household, and I know my family would agree. But my queen regularly demonstrates her capacity as a partner, mother, daughter, entrepreneur, leader and role model in ways that can only leave me in awe of her power, tenacity, talent and beauty. However, she is not immune to the impact of stress on her hormonal health. She has had to learn how to manage all of the roles she finds herself in to recoup her own energy, immune health and more. Through respect of her natural rhythm and hormonal support where necessary, Dr. Ashley Lucas has found the tools to continue her own mission and purpose. You can too.

The power of hormone optimization doesn't stop with menopause either. In fact, hormone therapy often gets simpler when the ovaries stop producing their own estrogen. Hormone optimization can look different on different women, but understanding your options is the starting point for success. So, Reason #1 why your hormones aren't working for you? You were never offered the best options of care in the first place. The traditional medical system fails to recognize the importance of hormone replacement and optimization for women as their hormones start to change in midlife. This can stop here and now.

To lay the groundwork for the rest of this book, let's review some basic terminology that can make the discussion of hormones challenging for consumers. Women have three primary sex hormones: estrogen, progesterone and testosterone. We will touch on each of these at length, but remember this for later. The estrogen that we will primarily be referring to is estradiol. Yes, there are others, but I'm trying to create as simple a discussion around hormones as I can, so we will only discuss estradiol. Progesterone is a powerful hormone that can be found as a replacement in two primary forms. Synthetic progestins and bioidentical micronized progesterone. Micronized progesterone is the natural form of the hormone, and unless otherwise stated, I am referring to oral micronized progesterone rather than artificial progestins when I say progesterone. You may also hear the term progestogen. This term encompasses both progesterone and progestins, and I won't use it in this text. Lastly, testosterone. When I say testosterone, I mean testosterone, not a special feminine form, but testosterone that you hear about as a "male" hormone. Women have testosterone too, just not as much as men but maybe more than you think!

There are also many confusing terms thrown out there when we start discussing replacement of hormones, and many authors and doctors are very particular about which one is used under certain circumstances. Let's clear this up so we are on the same page moving forward. Hormone Replacement Therapy (HRT) is a classically used term in the space of prescribing hormones for women. Recent publications have criticized authors for using this term because it doesn't really describe the goal of hormone optimization either before or after menopause. Perimenopausal women are often not "replacing" but optimizing hormones. Sometimes this process can use supplements, lifestyle changes or potentially hormones like testosterone and progesterone off-label to optimize but not fully replace natural hormone production. Postmenopausal women also may feel inadequately treated by "replacement" strategies because hormone therapy after menopause is often not attempting to completely replace premenopausal levels of all of the hormones nor are they generally trying to mimic natural hormone cycles.

Some authors prefer the term "Menopausal Hormone Therapy" (MHT). This term is more specific to the goal of treating menopause symptoms with hormones. I don't prefer this term for our approach because we are not simply treating the symptoms of menopause. We look at hormones as a tool to maximize health for as long as possible or "healthspan." MHT, in my opinion, is a shortsighted view of optimized hormone therapy and unlikely to provide adequate dosing to truly provide all of the potential benefits of hormone therapy.

Bioidentical Hormone Replacement Therapy (BHRT) is also a popular term indicating specific forms of hormone replacement that are "bioidentical." We will discuss this in detail near the end of the book. You may also see "estrogen therapy" indicating estrogen-only therapy, "combined therapy" indicating estrogen and some form of progesterone in combination, and lastly, testosterone replacement therapy (TRT), which would indicate testosterone-alone therapy. Moving forward, I will simply use the term HRT to indicate replacement of hormones from outside of the body. We will dive into specific forms and routes of replacement near the end of the text.

Throughout this book, we will review the maze of hormone optimization and replacement options, discussing the pros and cons of each. My goal is to empower you to make choices that align with your individual health goals and needs. We will review in depth the often-overstated risks and many misconceptions held by both patients and doctors. We will discuss the unique role of all three primary sex hormones (estrogen, progesterone and testosterone) for women. This book is a testament to my belief that every woman deserves access to the information and care necessary to thrive during this transformative season of life. The landscape of hormones is challenging for both patients and doctors. However, I see a revolution stirring in women and their care. Women deserve to know the truth and deserve to be treated with equality. Conversations around hormones seem hard, but they don't have to be. All it takes is the right perspective, knowledge and admission of and subsequent removal of bias. Again, Reason #1 that your hormones aren't working for you? The system has prevented you from pursuing your optimal self.

A final note before we begin. This book is about hormones and hormone optimization through dose, route and form of hormones. I will not spend much time discussing nutrition, gut health, exercise, stress management, connection, supplements or anything else that relates directly or indirectly to hormones, not because these things aren't critically important, but because I desperately want to get this information out and to do an exhaustive review to write a complete text is not possible with my current schedule! Hopefully in the future, you'll see a comprehensive text from me on these topics that I love, but for now, I'll stick to hormones themselves.

REASON #2

NOT USING ESTROGEN DUE TO FEAR OF BREAST CANCER AND BLOOD CLOTS

Estrogen is without a doubt the most talked about and researched of the three primary sex hormones, but there is still so much confusion and fear around it. To help you understand the controversy and position that I've taken, I need to give you a little background on historical estrogen therapy, what happened 20 years ago and what's happened since. Before the early 2000s, estrogen was prescribed for women often and without the shaming and negative connotation that often accompanies a prescription today.

Women used to be supported in their pursuit of relieving the symptoms of menopause as well as their health in perimenopause and beyond without criticism of wanting to use "dangerous hormones." Unfortunately, there were also practitioners who were using it inappropriately and making claims about heart health and longevity that had limited evidence to support them. This led to a need for good research to be conducted, and money flooded into research to answer the question, "Does estrogen indeed improve cardiovascular health and longevity?"

There were several studies that were conducted and published during the 90's and early 2000's. None more famous and impactful than the Women's Health Initiative (WHI). The WHI was a massive study that included four different intervention trials. Overall, it included over 160,000 participants and cost over $625,000,000! The angle the researchers took on hormones was to look at two specific groups: (1.) women without a uterus on estrogen-only therapy, and (2.) women with a uterus on combined estrogen and progestin therapy. Notice I used the word progestin there, not progesterone! The estrogen used in this study was a synthetic estrogen synthesized from horse's urine and given orally. It has lost market share but is still used today and is called either Conjugated Equine Estrogen (CEE) or the brand name Premarin® . The progestin used was Medroxyprogesterone Acetate (MPA) also known by the brand name, Provera® . Both oral, Premarin and Provera were popular at the time and were easy to prescribe and take as the combo drug PremPro.

Both study groups were primarily designed to show the potential benefit of HRT for heart health. Interestingly, both studies were stopped early but NOT for the same reason. The combined therapy group had 8,506 women randomized either to HRT or to a placebo (Rossouw, 2002). The study ran for an average exposure of 5.2 years before being terminated. The study was terminated due to concerns over increased risk from the HRT, specifically the development of invasive breast cancer. The data available at the time of termination was analyzed and the results published in July of 2002. The headlines, interpretations and conclusions made from this single publication changed the course of hormone replacement across the world at the time, and the impact is still reflected in prescribing patterns today. The takeaway message was clear: Hormone replacement increases the risk of breast cancer and very few women should be on estrogen therapy. I was in medical school during the years following this publication, and I clearly remember this message. I was guided to be on board with the anti-hormone bandwagon and taught that other options for symptoms of menopause should be considered. I did not have the critical thinking and research evaluation skills then that I do now.

After publishing a handful of peer-reviewed articles and book chapters and spending a decade on the research committee of an orthopedic organization, I have learned how to interpret data for myself. Now, when I look at the 2002 publication from the WHI, I understand why they did what they did, but I am appalled at the failure of the clinical physicians to understand the true message that should have been received! Let me explain.

The 2002 publication from the Women's Health Initiative clearly shows the statistical analysis of the data. When we look at data from prospective (looking forward) intervention trials, risk is often delivered in a "hazard ratio" (HR). Meaning that the risk of developing the effect or event in question is higher or lower than the placebo group. When the HR is >1, there is increased risk; and when it's <1, there is decreased risk or protection from an event. However, we also have to look at the "confidence interval" (CI). The CI is used to measure the precision of the HR. It is represented by a range of numbers. When the confidence interval includes the number 1, the HR is not statistically significant. When the range is completely above or below 1, the HR IS statistically significant. When a CI includes or crosses 1.0 and the result is deemed NOT statistically significant, clinical decision making comes into play. Statistical significance means that statistically, the effect we are seeing is not likely due to chance. Just because something is statistically significant, it doesn't mean that it is clinically significant. Meaning, it may not change how we treat patients. When something is nearly statistically significant, we call it a "trend" toward significance. Trends are still important; but generally, we don't make clinical changes without further evidence from a trend toward significance in a single study. Understanding that detail is critical here. While large studies are great at showing us risk and rare events with an intervention, we do have to be careful not to over extrapolate data into clinical practice. Large studies can show subtle signals that may not help us treat patients in real clinical scenarios. This can be challenging, but let's run through the WHI data to demonstrate how important these points are in interpreting a study like this.

First, let's look at the protective effects of the combined therapy group. They were looking primarily at heart attack and heart disease deaths (Coronary Heart Disease (CHD)), however, the secondary endpoints were cases of invasive breast cancer, endometrial cancer, colon cancer, fragility fractures and blood clot related events like pulmonary embolism (PE) and stroke as well as death due to other causes. Again, near and dear to my heart are fragility fractures, so let's start with hip fractures. There was a Hazard Ratio (HR) of 0.66 with a Confidence Interval (CI) of 0.43–0.92. That means that we can say there was a 44% reduction in hip fracture risk in the combined therapy group! The CI is all below 1, so it is statistically significant! Additionally, they report the actual number of fractures in each group, which helps us determine clinical significance. Colon cancer numbers were similar with an HR of 0.63 (47% reduction in risk) and a CI of 0.43–0.92, all under 1, so it's statistically significant.

Now, let's look at invasive breast cancer diagnosis. They reported an HR of 1.26 (26% increase) and CI of 1.00–1.59. Remember what I said about the CI crossing 1? This finding does not reach statistical significance! Is it clinically relevant? Maybe. The study was designed to stop if certain safety thresholds were met, and this trend toward significance crossed that threshold. What does it mean clinically? Well, they report that per 10,000 patient years, there would be 8 more cases of invasive breast cancer diagnosed in those on combined HRT. Is that clinically relevant? Some would say yes, some say no. We don't need to debate that here because there was another study that helps us find our way through this mess. This second study was also from the WHI.

The second WHI publication was looking at the group taking Premarin (CEE) alone because they had undergone a hysterectomy and no longer had a uterus. Because the estrogen used in each trial was the same, this publication can help us differentiate what, if any, risk was likely coming from the progestin component of the combined HRT. This group was stopped early too but not for the same reason as listed in the first publication. Their statistical analysis identified a pattern of concern, not for risk but for failure to meet the primary endpoint of showing CHD benefit. So, the study was stopped, and the data was reported in 2004 (Anderson, 2004). They again showed similar improvement in colon cancer reduction as well as hip fracture, but the biggest difference was in the statistics around invasive breast cancer! The HR for breast cancer was 0.77 with a CI of 0.59–1.01. This shows a trend toward protection of breast cancer with CEE of 23%. Again, a 23% reduction in invasive breast cancer risk. However, we have to remember that the CI needs to make it below one to be statistically significant, but the trend here can't be ignored. They openly state this in their conclusion as well by saying that the "possible reduction in breast cancer risk requires further investigation."

What's so compelling to me about comparing these data is how similar the increased risk is in the first study with combined therapy to the decreased risk in the second study with estrogen alone. Yet, the sentiment was unchanged in the clinical population that HRT causes breast cancer and that we should avoid estrogen therapy and use "safer" treatments for symptoms of menopause, like antidepressants. Women were faced with an impossible decision to ignore their doctors and seek treatment from those willing to prescribe HRT or suffer in silence. So many did the latter. I see them now in my practice with osteoporosis, sarcopenia and regret.

Now, 20 years later, there have been numerous studies published reanalyzing these data and demonstrating the potential flaws of the design around the WHI as well as different statistical approaches that demonstrate different results. Textbooks could be written on this data, but a recent 20-year follow-up publication sums it up well. This publication reviews all of the studies published on long-term follow-up on the clinical trials performed in the WHI (Manson, 2024). Specifically, regarding invasive breast cancer, here's what happened. The statistically insignificant findings in the 2002 publication did eventually reach significance, and that risk persisted in long-term follow-up. Again, a damning publication for progestins, not estrogen. The 2004 estrogen-only group also reached statistical significance in long-term follow-up, and that protection from breast cancer also persisted. Seems like the disparity just kept growing between the treatment groups. Again, the guilty party here should have been the progestin from the beginning. Not only does this long-term data support it, but multiple other studies do as well. Consider the following:

- A 2023 bench study showed that progestins upregulate gene expression for cancer at MUCH higher rates than micronized progesterone (Lalitkumar, 2023).
- A 2017 Swedish cohort study on 290,000 women demonstrated increased breast cancer risk with combined HRT but noted that progestin use carries the majority of that risk (Simin, 2017).
- A 2022 UK cohort study on 43,000 breast cancer cases demonstrated that only progestin use was associated with an increased risk of breast cancer development (28% increased risk). Neither estrogen nor micronized progesterone carried this same risk (Abenheim, 2022).
- The initially damning Million Women Study showed a massive, 100% increase in breast cancer risk with the use of progestin therapy (Beral, 2003).

The list goes on and on, but I think you get the picture. Progestins are devious and should be avoided, especially when there is a suitable and more natural alternative. As mentioned previously, micronized progesterone is safer, and according to a 2022 meta analysis, either equal to or better than progestins in regard to (Graham, 2022):

- Preventing endometrial hyperplasia.
- Preventing breast cancer diagnosis.
- Preventing cardiovascular disease.
- Preventing age related cognitive decline.
- Preventing fractures.

Additionally, these authors explored estradiol alone versus CEE and found that estradiol:

- Reduced the risk of blood clots.
- Better protects against age-related cognitive decline.
- Better protects against fractures.

Looks like some alternatives to the CEE and MPA can provide a safer alternative to the popular HRT at the time.

Over the last 20 years, compelling evidence for the use of estradiol continued to be published. Two areas that deserve further discussion are breast cancer diagnosis and death from breast cancer. We will start with breast cancer deaths. This is a delicate point to make because I don't wish a breast cancer diagnosis on anyone. However, breast cancer is a common diagnosis, and as such, the impact of being on HRT at the time of diagnosis is an important impact to explore. Fortunately, a 2016 Finnish study sought to explore that impact directly. Turns out that the HRT users, either with estradiol alone or in combination with a progestin, that were diagnosed with breast cancer were less likely to die as a result of that breast cancer (Mikkola, 2016). Estradiol alone through any form demonstrated up to a 54% reduction in risk of death from breast cancer. The benefit was reduced with the addition of progestins to estrogen as low as a 12% reduction with some formulations.

There are two primary explanations provided in the article. First, as I stated above, women on HRT were more likely to receive screening for breast cancer on a regular basis. Secondly, the cancers themselves were more likely to have "benign histological features and favorable biomarkers." Ultimately, their cancers were identified earlier and were more likely to be survivable. Cancer treatment is a difficult topic and outside of the scope of this book. What to do with hormone replacement during the subsequent cancer battle is a contentious and challenging conversation with strong emotions from both sides of the argument for and against HRT in the face of breast cancer. I hope to discuss this in depth on our YouTube channels, The Dr. Doug Show and PEMA-BioIdentical, in the future. See your reader resources page for links to the YouTube channels and other resources on this topic.

The last point we need to make here is around the continued signal that estrogen may contribute to a breast cancer diagnosis. I love our freedom of speech, but I get frustrated by the very strong statements some influencers and doctors make regarding hormones and risk. I don't believe hormones are without risk, but we need to understand what the risk really is. To say that estrogen doesn't cause breast cancer is a strong statement, and from my research, a true statement. BUT to say that estrogen isn't involved in breast cancer would be misleading. There are too many studies that continue to show an increased risk of diagnosis of breast cancer during HRT. Some of the larger studies (like the Million Women Study from the UK and the WHI) have open access data banks, which have been analyzed statistically and papers published with adjusted data that show there is no statistically significant increase in risk, BUT even those papers still show a trend toward risk (Shapiro, 2012).

So, how do I reconcile that with my patients? I look at it like this. Breast cancer is often hormone receptor positive. Breast cancer is also relatively common, with 1 out of 8 women in the US developing breast cancer in their lifetime. If a hormone sensitive cancer develops while a woman is on HRT, it may impact the growth. This could lead to an increase in diagnosed cases during any set amount of time in a study. Breast cancers often take months or years to grow large enough to be identified on mammograms, even with newer 3D technology. If HRT could provoke more rapid growth and a study was carried out for 5 or 10 years, it makes sense that we would see more cancers in a specified time frame versus those not on HRT.

So, is estrogen the CAUSE of breast cancer? No. Does it make it grow faster? Possibly. But as we've demonstrated already, having been on HRT reduces the risk of death from breast cancer that would have occurred anyway. Additionally, estrogen has also been shown to stabilize cancers, especially with adequate progesterone. This is the risk we need to discuss with our patients as they consider HRT. This is a VERY different conversation than most of my patients have reported to me that they had when initially considering HRT with less knowledgeable providers.

One last risk to discuss stemming from the WHI, and then we will move on. HRT has been associated with an increased risk of blood clot related events, stroke, deep vein thrombosis (DVT) and pulmonary embolism (PE). We saw this clearly in the WHI, and it was picked up in other studies too. This risk is EASY to avoid by simply understanding the role of progestins in the development of blood clots and the role of different routes of estrogen. Progestins are well-known to increase the risk of blood clot alone. We see this in oral birth control pills, and the same is true for combined formulations of HRT (Roach,

2015). Micronized progesterone does not carry this same risk as discussed above (Panay, 2023). Additionally, oral estradiol itself has been implicated in an increased risk of blood clot. This is controversial, but rather than spending your time arguing the two sides, we can simply show that switching to a topical formulation either through patch or cream mitigates that risk (Vinogradova, 2019).

So, now we have demonstrated that well-designed HRT can be provided with no increased risk of developing breast cancer, dying from breast cancer or suffering a stroke, DVT or PE. Reason #2 your HRT is failing you? You simply never started estrogen because of a misunderstanding of risk. I hope you can see now that many of the commonly held risks are overstated and that many more women should be able to start HRT if they could have the right risk/benefit conversation.

REASON #3

NOT USING PROGESTERONE BECAUSE YOU DON'T HAVE A UTERUS

Progesterone has historically only been given to women as a part of hormone replacement therapy to protect the uterine lining from "hypertrophy" or overgrowth, which increases the risk of endometrial (uterine) cancer.

While important, this single use of progesterone misses the bigger picture and possibilities of this critical hormone for women. Additionally, progesterone has become synonymous with the synthetic counterparts, progestins, which we have already seen have very different risk profiles. Understanding the benefits of bioidentical micronized progesterone (MP) and the differences between MP and progestins will be critical to your hormone replacement success story! Unfortunately, we won't see a lot of data here. Because progesterone has been relegated to the support character for estrogen, it is rarely studied alone. However, some truth and opportunity for optimization is available in research to share. Clinically, I have been using progesterone in unique ways that I'd love to share with you as well. This hormone has many potential benefits that are often underappreciated. Micronized progesterone could be a key missing element for women not feeling optimized on their HRT!

First, a little history. Progesterone has been available medically since the 1930s, and the synthetic progestins became available in the 1950s. At the time, the progestins offered superior absorption and effectiveness over the original bioidentical version until the technology to "micronize" the latter became available in the 1970s. That delay in technology to improve absorption allowed the progestins to gain a foothold within the pharmaceutical industry and become the standard of care in HRT.

In premenopausal women, progesterone and estrogen balance each other cyclically with each having a window of dominance before the cycle starts over again. The back and forth between progesterone and estrogen allows for each to play its unique role in the body. Changes occur on a cellular, receptor and even epigenetic level with the regular cycling of these hormones. This is seen very clearly with one of my passion topics, bone health. Cyclic and natural estrogen withdrawal around day 14 of the menstrual cycle provokes increased osteoclast activity. These cells break down bone, which we need to do in order to make new bone. Progesterone, which rises after the estrogen fall, stimulates the bone-building cells (osteoblasts) to fill in the space that has been made by the osteoclasts (Prior, 2018).

This seesaw rhythm allows for the maintenance of strong bones until menopause or loss of hormonal balance, whichever occurs first. In combination with estrogen, we see clear reduction in fracture risk, at least initially (Rossouw, 2002). There is also evidence to support the protective effect of progesterone on breast cancer development (Formby, 1998). In fact, some authors strongly encourage timing surgeries for breast cancer removal, like lumpectomy and mastectomy, around the luteal phase of the menstrual cycle because the presence of progesterone reduces the risk of recurrence and improves outcomes (Chaudhry, 2006), Again, demonstrating that the seesaw rhythm of progesterone and estrogen has therapeutic implications.

Estrogen is known for its beneficial effects on night sweats and hot flashes, but don't be so sure that progesterone doesn't play a role as well! In a small randomized controlled trial, oral micronized progesterone at 300 mg reduced symptoms of hot flashes and night sweats more than a placebo (Hitchcock,

2012). For women that are not candidates for estrogen therapy, there may be an off-label opportunity to leverage the lower risk counterpart in MP. This may be in part due to progesterone's known impact on blood vessel health. Progesterone is thought to promote vasodilation of arteries and improve the function of the artery lining called the endothelium (Santos, 2014). This could result in improved blood pressure and possibly reduced risk of blood clot, especially when compared to their synthetic counterpart. They may also play a role in cholesterol function and improve lipid biomarkers. There is conflicting data on this topic, but all of the prospective studies that have been done consistently show no harm to the cardiovascular system and no increased risk associated with replacement of progesterone as MP.

One recent study that came out as this manuscript was finished made headlines for claiming increased risk of MP compared to progestin (Baik, 2024). While the big picture takeaway from this large retrospective study was that HRT is protective of many chronic diseases associated with aging, it was the first study to make the claim that progestins were more protective than MP. Although a large study, it still suffers from the potential bias and weaknesses of a retrospective cohort. Additionally, studies like this one look at prescriptions for medications, not whether someone is actually taking the medication. There is no accountability for compliance. While the authors try to control for other factors that could lead to erroneous conclusions, we must match these data with prospective, RCT data to identify clinically relevant risk and causation. No prospective study has shown similar results, and therefore, we should only use this new study as a tool to make a hypothesis. And I maintain that MP is safe and likely protective of the arterial endothelial cells of the arteries and elsewhere in the body.

Progesterone also impacts the brain and other neurological structures throughout a woman's lifespan when replaced appropriately (Schumacher, 2008). Progesterone is thought to help promote the growth and repair the lining of nerves within the central nervous system. Destruction of the myelin sheath can be part of the process of neurodegeneration leading to dementia. Additionally, when orally delivered, progesterone is metabolized into allopregnanolone, which acts through GABA receptors to promote a calming effect on the brain. This is part of the powerful impact we see on sleep with oral progesterone replacement in those that need it. Sleep is such an important topic when it comes to perimenopause and menopause hormonal changes. While all three primary sex hormones play a role in optimizing sleep, oral progesterone replacement has the most reliable and often immediate effect on sleep for my patients.

Progesterone clearly does more than just balance the lining of the uterus as many doctors would tell their patients. It plays a role in the health of the brain, heart, breast, bones and more. I strongly recommend progesterone replacement for women with symptoms of progesterone deficiency or for health optimization overall. Progesterone can also be a powerful tool for women with naturally cycling estrogen and symptoms of estrogen dominance, such as bloating, tender breasts, erratic mood swings and heavy menstrual flow to name a few. Perimenopausal hormone optimization often requires cyclic MP replacement. For postmenopausal women, the symptoms can be deceptive. I find that postmenopausal women without a uterus who are on estrogen-only therapy still struggle with sleep and may also notice brain fog and decreased cognitive function. My recommendation to those patients is to consider off-label oral micronized progesterone, and frequently we see big improvements.

A warning about topical progesterone. There are some advocates out there for topical progesterone over oral. It's also popular because it can be obtained without the hassle of a physician's prescription. While good-quality micronized progesterone cream can deliver adequate progesterone systemically, it's hard to measure. It's not carried through the bloodstream, like estradiol is or like MP is, when delivered orally. As a result, it's difficult to know if we are supplying adequate progesterone to protect the uterus from hypertrophy. Not only is this potentially dangerous, it also concerns me that if we aren't seeing adequate progesterone with topical administration for the uterus, it is also not likely adequate elsewhere. I'm not opposed to topical application, BUT very clear guidelines have to be established around safety if a menstrual cycle is not being used to verify if adequate progesterone is present. We will discuss physiologic and rhythmic HRT later in this text.

Another issue with progesterone to consider is quality. While oral MP is available commercially and carries FDA approval for use in the US, there are two issues I run up against when prescribing progesterone through commercial pharmacies. First, it's only available in 100 mg and 200 mg doses. Some women don't tolerate these specific doses and do better with 150, 250 or more. Because MP is delivered in capsules, it's difficult to use commercially available products to hit these in-between doses. Secondly, commercial products are made with peanut oil, glycerin, lecithin, titanium dioxide, Yellow no. 10 and Red no. 40. Why commercial products need to be made with such garbage ingredients is beyond me!

We prefer to compound micronized progesterone to avoid these toxins, hit the dose our patients need and generally use an extended-release formula, which is also not available commercially. Reason #3 why your HRT may be failing you? You aren't on progesterone at all or don't have the right dose, quality product or route of progesterone.

REASON #4

IGNORING STRESS AND ADRENAL HEALTH

Testosterone is most frequently discussed in the realm of men's health. Over the next two chapters, I want to discuss the ins and outs of testosterone for women both naturally and through replacement. In both men and women, testosterone can be made naturally in three different areas: reproductive glands (testes and ovaries), adrenal glands and "peripheral conversion" of precursor hormones.

In men, testosterone is made primarily in the testes, 95%. About 5% is made in the adrenal glands and peripheral tissues through hormone precursors, like androstenedione and dehydroepiandrosterone (DHEA). In women, there is stark contrast: 25% of testosterone is made in the ovaries, 25% directly in the adrenal glands and 50% made in the peripheral tissues. So, 75% of a woman's testosterone comes directly from the adrenal glands or from precursors made in the adrenal glands. This is good news for postmenopausal women because that means that 75% of production of testosterone is still possible after ovarian failure (menopause) has occurred.

I believe this is one reason why symptoms of menopause seem to be so much more pronounced now than historically. I will demonstrate later just how many of the symptoms of menopause may be from testosterone deficiency, but for now, let's just assume that testosterone plays a role. Imagine then if a woman going through menopause still had adequate testosterone. Yes, estrogen deficiency symptoms may still occur, but they would be blunted by the presence of testosterone, AND they would still see low levels of estrogen from aromatization of testosterone to estrogen that may additionally reduce or eliminate symptoms altogether. Testosterone deficiency may play a role here, and the root of this comes from the adrenal glands and their health. Before we discuss replacement, let's talk about how important natural production can be!

The production of cortisol and adrenal testosterone is intricately linked through their precursor substances and the regulatory mechanisms that control their synthesis. Both cortisol and adrenal testosterone is synthesized from cholesterol, but their production is tightly regulated by adrenocorticotropic hormone (ACTH) from the pituitary gland. Under normal conditions, ACTH stimulates the adrenal cortex to produce both cortisol and testosterone in a balanced manner. However, during periods of prolonged stress, the demand for cortisol increases significantly. When cortisol goes up, sex hormone levels start to go down. In times of chronic stress, testosterone levels can be reduced in three ways!

First, the body prioritizes cortisol production to cope with the stress, utilizing more of the common precursors for its synthesis. This shift can lead to a relative decrease in the production of adrenal testosterone, a phenomenon known as "cortisol steal" or "pregnenolone steal." The mechanism involves the diversion of pregnenolone, a common precursor for all adrenal steroids, towards the production of cortisol at the expense of testosterone. The increased demand for cortisol affects the adrenal gland's capacity to produce androgens. The reduced androgen production capacity of the adrenal glands will profoundly impact women more than men because of the disparity in location of testosterone production.

Second, cortisol itself will negatively impact androgen production. Chronic stress that leads to chronically elevated cortisol can have numerous negative downstream effects. Chronic elevation of cortisol can suppress the secretion of GnRH (gonadotropin-releasing hormone) from the brain.

Since GnRH is essential for stimulating the production of sex hormones in the pituitary gland, its suppression can lead to decreased levels of LH (luteinizing hormone) and FSH (follicle-stimulating hormone), which in turn can lower the stimulation of the ovaries to produce testosterone. That remaining 25% of production for women is then also impacted by stress.

The third way that stress reduces testosterone is through SHBG (sex hormone-binding globulin). High levels of cortisol can lead to an increase in the production of SHBG, the protein that binds to testosterone, making it unavailable for use by the body. This effectively reduces the amount of bioavailable or free testosterone. There may also be a negative effect on peripheral conversion as well, but this mechanism is not clearly understood.

Testosterone deficiency in women is then uniquely associated with the societal stresses that puts undue strain on the adrenal glands, gut and more. Running a practice that measures adrenal function in all patients, I can tell you that adrenal dysfunction is rampant, and low levels of DHEA and testosterone are strongly associated with it. Therefore, women who have any amount of adrenal dysfunction from stress will see lowering levels of testosterone and potentially accompanying progesterone and estrogen dysfunction. Chronic stress truly will impact women's hormones more than men's as a result of this organ production balancing act.

To make matters worse, we also have a testosterone deficiency epidemic in men. This book isn't about men, BUT hear me out because women's testosterone is under attack from more than one direction! Men's testosterone levels have been declining steadily over the last several decades (Travison, 2007). One leading theory behind the decline points to environmental influences, particularly the increased exposure to endocrine-disrupting chemicals (EDCs). These substances, found in plastics, pesticides, and personal care products, can mimic or interfere with the body's hormonal processes. EDCs like phthalates and bisphenol A (BPA) have been linked to lowered testosterone levels, suggesting a direct connection between increased environmental pollution and hormonal disturbances.

Modern lifestyle changes also play a crucial role. Factors such as decreased physical activity and a poor diet have been implicated in the decline of testosterone. Obesity, in particular, poses a significant risk, as excess visceral body fat can convert testosterone into estrogen, further reducing available testosterone. Men don't see the same impact of chronic stress on testosterone production in the adrenal glands, BUT the chronically elevated cortisol levels can also suppress the sex organ's ability to produce testosterone in men as it does in women. Testosterone appears to be exquisitely sensitive to sleep disturbance and perceived stress. Dietary changes over the years, including increased consumption of ultra-processed foods and reduced intake of essential nutrients like zinc, may contribute to hormonal imbalances as well. The same combination of environmental factors and stress have decimated women's testosterone production and sets the stage for greater challenges through midlife and beyond than ever before.

It's not surprising then that we find a signal of this dysfunction in the literature. Indeed, there is evidence to demonstrate that women's levels of testosterone drop starting early in adulthood. Statistically, women will have half the circulating testosterone at 40 as they did at 21 (Zumoff, 1995). That publication was almost 30 years ago, and if hormone dysfunction in women is mirroring that from men, it's likely much worse now. So, Reason #4 that your HRT is failing you is that either you are on testosterone and are relying too heavily on this tool OR your adrenal glands, lifestyle and supplement recommendations need work!

REASON #5

IGNORING TESTOSTERONE

In women, testosterone is less frequently discussed than estrogen. Testosterone is often misunderstood, and as a result often either under- or even sometimes over-utilized. There is a lot of confusion here, so let me try to shed some light on the myths and misconceptions around the androgen testosterone.

While it's true that women have less testosterone than men, what may surprise you is that women should have more testosterone than they do estrogen by volume. In fact, when adjusted for units, a woman will have 5–10 times more testosterone than estrogen at any point in her life (Glaser, 2013) (fig 1). It may seem then that this should be the most important hormone for women, but remember what I said in the chapter above. Women can still make optimal testosterone after menopause, and volume of sex hormone doesn't necessarily equal importance of sex hormone.

So, the tricky question is when we see perceived testosterone deficiency by either symptoms or lab biomarkers, we have to ask ourselves, "Is it adrenal dysfunction? Precursor deficiency? True testosterone deficiency? Or imbalanced estrogen and progesterone?" This nuance is critical because as you'll see below, much of the evidence around testosterone is treatment with testosterone alone. Rarely do we see an intervention that optimizes estradiol, progesterone and healthy adrenal function while providing precursors for natural testosterone production or all three primary hormones together in concert. In our practice, we have been using testosterone replacement as a tool for years and have extensive experience in this challenging gray area. Let me walk you through what we've learned.

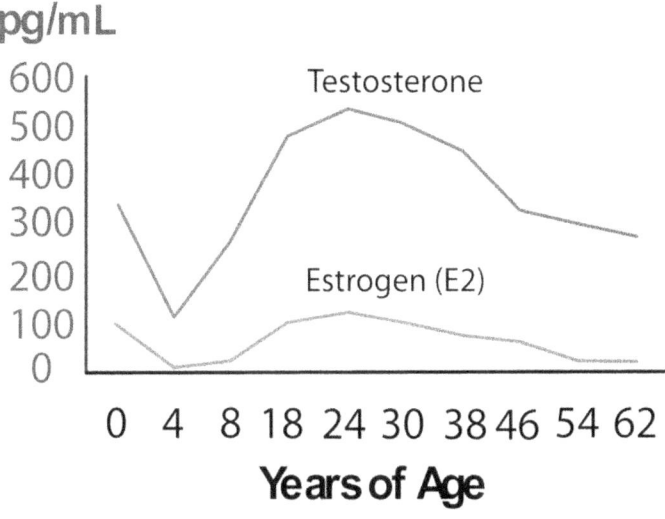

Figure 1: Demonstrates the average testosterone and estradiol levels in women throughout her lifespan when adjusted to the same units in pg/mL.

Before we dig into the research on testosterone, first let me explain the relationship with these sometimes-confusing terms. Testosterone is one hormone of a group of hormones called androgens. This group consists of testosterone, dihydrotestosterone (DHT), androstenedione and dehydroepiandrosterone (DHEA). As we walk through this research, you'll see the term "androgen deficiency" and "testosterone deficiency." Many authors use these terms interchangeably, but there is some nuance to consider. We should consider testosterone through the lens of androgen deficiency, and by doing so, we open more treatment options than simply testosterone replacement alone. You'll see why this is important.

As mentioned earlier, research and medical care for women has historically been suboptimal. The history of testosterone replacement in women is not just another example of this, but I think it should be considered a medical tragedy for the extent at which this hormone and androgens in general have been ignored and sidelined. The majority of research on testosterone in women is centered around the diagnosis of "Hypoactive Sexual Desire Disorder" (HSDD). This psychiatric disorder is defined by "a lack of sexual desire or interest in sexual activity, which can lead to personal distress or interpersonal difficulties." My patients confirm my suspicion, which is that this topic rarely comes up in their traditional medical practitioner's office, and when it does, they are not likely to do anything about it. There is a recommendation from physician organizations for short-term testosterone therapy under these circumstances, BUT even if a willing doctor wanted to prescribe testosterone in the US, there is no commercial product for women to be prescribed. This leaves the willing provider with the option of prescribing something they may feel more comfortable with, like an antidepressant, do nothing at all, prescribe a product designed for men at a lower dose or use a compounding pharmacy, which they may not be comfortable with either. To make matters more complicated, testosterone is listed as a Schedule III controlled substance by the FDA, which puts it in the same risk class as known addictive and harmful drugs like the infamous narcotic painkillers. Many physicians prescribe testosterone with fear of criticism and oversight by medical boards and medical associations, and when faced with this conundrum, alternatives to testosterone start to look pretty good, regardless of their effectiveness for patients. Remember too that most physicians are not trained in lifestyle optimization and over-the-counter supplementation, so these recommendations are rare as well.

Before we get to the actual proven benefits of testosterone in women, let's further explore the travesty of the failure of the medical establishment to adequately explore testosterone therapy in women. Doctors are not educated on hormone replacement in general but certainly not on testosterone in women. We physicians are left to explore these therapies on our own and to do additional training where needed to help our patients. When I first started learning about hormone replacement in women, I remember quite vividly reading the recommendations from the endocrine society about testosterone. This society is the go-to organization for all things hormones for most traditional medical doctors. Their recommendations set the tone for treatment nationwide. Here is a portion of their recommendations from a 2006 review paper on the topic from when I was in training (Wierman, 2006).

"We (The Endocrine Society) continue to recommend against making a diagnosis of androgen deficiency syndrome in healthy women because there is a lack of a well-defined syndrome, and data correlating androgen levels with specific signs or symptoms are unavailable." A more updated internationally accepted consensus statement goes on to say that "the only evidence-based indication for testosterone therapy for women is for the treatment of HSDD." They did not identify sufficient data to support the use of testosterone for treatment of any other symptom or clinical condition, or for disease prevention (Davis, 2019).

Both of these statements get further into specifics which effectively pigeonhole physicians into having to diagnose HSDD in order to recommend testosterone therapy for women, which most do not seem willing to do, especially when there is no commercial product to prescribe anyway. What is remarkable to me about these statements is the "lack of a well-defined syndrome" comment. What they're saying is that because there are no obvious symptoms of an androgen deficiency, replacement should not be recommended.

No obvious symptoms? Wow, my practice specializing in osteoporosis provides me with lots of evidence to the contrary. In fact, when we look at aging in general, we can see some obvious symptoms that would benefit from androgens that are well-defined and badly need to be addressed. I'm in a unique position to see the ravages of androgen deficiency in women's health in the perimenopause and postmenopausal time frames. Through my practice focusing on osteoporosis (Optimal Human Health MD (OHH)) and my platform specifically focusing on hormone replacement (PEMA BioIdentical), we serve hundreds of women that have developed sarcopenia (loss of muscle mass) and osteoporosis (loss of bone mass and quality). These women very frequently also demonstrate other signs and symptoms of androgen deficiency. Why do I see it and others don't? In this regard, I'm not special. The symptoms are just hiding in plain sight, and differentiating them from other sex hormone deficiencies can be challenging if you don't know where to look.

Why this hasn't been studied historically seems to be rooted in the discrimination of women in medical research and because testosterone is generally only discussed in the face of sexual dysfunction in "older women." I use quotes here to indicate that I'm not defining what "older" means chronologically. I actually see the need for testosterone in what I would consider younger women in their 30s and even 20s! The reason why "older" is important to consider is that our society doesn't like to talk about sex in the context of older women. Men's sexual appetite and performance is considered important at nearly all ages, but women are only glorified sexually as young adults, and interest in their sexual needs fades in society as they age. We are quietly and subconsciously told that it's okay for men to want to have a strong libido regardless of age, but women's libido should only be considered and discussed when they are "young." What I want to stress as we move forward is that androgen deficiency isn't just about sex and desire. Many women express to me that androgen replacement or optimization can improve their feelings of self-worth, self-confidence and help them with the ability to engage in intimacy regardless of the desire for intercourse. Beyond all of the intimacy and sex talk lies the bigger picture of the benefits of androgens which reach far beyond the libido. Fortunately, the last few decades have seen plenty of research to demonstrate what testosterone deficiency really is and where to look.

Studies on menopause are very interesting to me. First, for a process that every woman will go through should she live long enough, menopause seems very poorly studied! There are large gaps in the body of knowledge in menopause, but studies on symptoms and symptom relief have really caught my attention. One such study I'd like to direct our attention to in regard to androgen therapy is a 2011 prospective cohort study on 300 symptomatic women using a tool called the Menopause Rating Scale (MRS). They sought to study the symptoms of menopause and perimenopause with exposure to testosterone specifically (Glaser, 2011). The MRS is a standardized scale that is used to assess the severity of menopause symptoms. The symptoms listed in the scale are:

Vasomotor Symptoms
- Hot flashes
- Night sweats
- Sweating

Heart Discomfort
- Heart palpitations
- Unusual sensations in the chest

Sleep Problems
- Difficulty sleeping
- Insomnia
- Poor quality sleep

Depressed Mood
- Feelings of sadness
- Lack of drive
- Mood swings

Irritability
- Feelings of agitation
- Nervousness
- Overly sensitive

Anxiety
- Inner tension
- Feelings of panic

Physical and Mental Exhaustion
- General tiredness
- Decreased energy levels

Sexual Problems
- Changes in desire
- Decreased satisfaction
- Discomfort during intercourse
- Vaginal dryness

Bladder Problems
- Urinary incontinence
- Increased frequency of urination

Joint and Muscular Discomfort
- Achiness
- Joint pain
- Muscular tension

They administered this tool to 300 women before and after testosterone therapy alone. This group involved both premenopausal and postmenopausal women and provides some incredible insight into the benefits of this type of therapy! This clinical study measured blood levels at the beginning of the trial for all symptomatic women, and while most did have low testosterone, some were in the upper third of the "normal." But a crucial point is that **ALL WERE WITHIN THE LAB REFERENCE RANGE.** This is critical to understand because, like men, when testosterone IS checked by a woman's doctor, so often their symptoms are dismissed because their labs are "normal." We run into this every day in our attempts to optimize our patients. Many times, the reference ranges for labs are statistical averages for the population at large. In a sick population or in the case of hormones in a postmenopausal population that naturally has lost them, the reference range is useless and may even include the number "0." To suggest that the lab-provided reference range should be our target misses the point of hormone optimization. Understanding what optimal values of hormones are requires an understanding of the concepts of healthspan.

Additionally, I applaud the authors of this study for using the blood test, free testosterone, rather than total testosterone alone in their methods and analysis. A common error for most doctors attempting to evaluate testosterone in blood is using total testosterone alone. Factors such as a woman's level of Sex Hormone Binding Globulin (SHBG) will dictate how much "active" or free testosterone is circulating in blood. Total testosterone should not be used alone because it is not directly correlated with levels of free testosterone! When these authors classified their participants, 87% of them had low free testosterone. A few had middle and upper-third free testosterone levels but clear symptoms of androgen deficiency and were included in the study.

Another consideration from this article is that premenopausal women and postmenopausal women exhibited different symptoms of androgen deficiency. Psychological complaints such as depressed mood, irritability and anxiety were higher in premenopausal women. Postmenopausal women were more likely to report "somatic" complaints, like hot flashes and vaginal dryness.

While I am grateful that this study was done, I don't agree that this therapy is optimal. My bias in training and practice has taught me that testosterone alone will fail to alleviate all of the symptoms just as estrogen and progesterone therapy alone will fail when testosterone levels are inadequate naturally. I believe that we should restore to a reasonable degree all three primary sex hormones to truly optimize a woman's hormones and health. This study does show the power of testosterone with improvement that was not just statistically significant but also clinically impressive with 60–74% improvement in EVERY category of the MRS. Those with the worst symptoms improved the most, but what I'd love to see is a comparison of the improvements to other interventions. While helpful, this study leaves many questions unanswered for me as a clinician.

I'd like to further explore and debunk the "lack of evidence" comment by the endocrine society. This is a common reason physicians will cite when they choose not to use androgens in practice, and they have plenty of support from societies like the endocrine society and others in choosing not to do so. However, there is good research on testosterone specifically in the sexual health and bone health spaces. This not only allows us the opportunity to see what the impact is but also helps to demonstrate safety, dosing and possible side effects of using testosterone replacement.

One of the largest sexual health studies on testosterone, the "Aphrodite" trial, was performed in 2008 on 814 women who carried a diagnosis of HSDD but were NOT on estrogen and progestin HRT. They were given a testosterone patch OR placebo (Davis, 2008). They looked at benefits of treatment for HSDD over 24 weeks and evaluated safety for up to 52 weeks with a subgroup evaluated for 2 years in total. The primary endpoint was an increase in 4-week frequency of satisfying sexual episodes. Additional endpoints included safety data around breast cancer, endometrial (uterine) hypertrophy with breakthrough bleeding, side effects and serum biomarkers of testosterone levels. The study demonstrated at 24 weeks that the highest dose of testosterone did, in fact, result in an increase in satisfying sexual encounters. Both low and high doses increased desire and decreased distress compared to placebo.

For many physicians, this study could be misunderstood and high doses of testosterone viewed as the only effective tool. However, baseline metrics in the study population showed that 50% of sexual encounters were satisfying. For a group with a diagnosis of HSDD, that's surprisingly high. After 24 weeks, the lower-dose group reported 65% of episodes to be satisfying and the higher-dose group 78%. Only the latter was statistically significant, but again, with a high starting point, that's not surprising. Questionnaires are notoriously inaccurate for topics like sexual frequency and satisfaction. Whenever a participant knows that their answers will be linked to their name and identifiable, answers seem to change. That may have played a role in the surprisingly high starting point and diminished the impact of testosterone therapy. My patients who experience symptoms of HSDD tell me that they have distress and dissatisfaction with nearly all sexual encounters for one reason or another, so again, 50% seems high for this population.

This study did a great job of looking at side effects, and because it was a large study with 2 years of follow-up and a placebo group, we can really see the placebo effect in action! If you aren't familiar with the placebo effect, let me quickly describe it. This is so important here! The placebo effect describes any changes associated with a placebo or fake intervention. Frequently, drug trials will use a capsule with an inert substance that should have no impact on the body. In this case, the placebo was a patch with no drug available for absorption. The placebo effect is important to consider because just like we can see false benefits with placebo, we can see false side effects too.

The side effects listed in this study included all things "androgenic" or coming from the androgen effect of testosterone. These include hair growth, hair loss, oily skin, acne, deepening of the voice and even genital/clitoral enlargement. These were graded as mild, moderate and severe. The abstract states that the higher-dose testosterone group had higher rates of androgenic events compared to placebo. Interestingly though when we explore the breakdown of these data, we see that only mild hair growth was statistically significantly higher. There were plenty of complaints by participants, but almost all of the complaints were higher or the same in the placebo group as compared to the higher-dose testosterone group. Additionally, they measured blood levels of total and free testosterone, and the levels in blood were not correlated to the frequency of side effects. What does that mean? It means that while I believe in measuring levels to understand absorption metrics and impact of dosing, we can't use levels alone to determine success in treatment or risk of side effects. In fact, the one participant that reported clitoral enlargement was in the lower-dose group not the higher-dose group. They did not report on any objective verification of the claimed anatomical change. Additionally, the placebo group reported MORE side effects, like hair loss and voice deepening, than the higher-dose testosterone group. A nice demonstration of the power of the mind. The women in the placebo group I'm sure honestly noticed these changes in themselves, but they were receiving no testosterone.

I support my patients doing their own research, but when they read over and over again that the therapy they may or may not be on could cause these concerning side effects, they may start to see those side effects in themselves. Where focus goes, energy flows. We are remarkable creatures that can create both positive and negative things in our lives! All of these possibilities have to be taken into consideration when optimizing hormones. Fortunately, the Aphrodite trial isn't the only study showing us potential benefits and side effects. A 2005 24-week RCT on 447 participants with three doses of testosterone patches compared to placebo showed very similar results (Braunstein, 2005). Additionally, the 2006 "INTIMATE" study and another study on surgically induced menopause in women with HSDD both studied testosterone in addition to traditional HRT with similarly compelling results (Shifren, 2006; Davis, 2006).

Testosterone is also well-studied in the bone health and osteoporosis space. This is actually where my interest in testosterone for women began. We have an entire program at OHH dedicated to identifying the causes of bone loss and reversing those causes as well as osteoporosis naturally in most people. If you are interested in this topic, please consider my book, *The Osteoporosis Breakthrough*. Links are available on the Resources page. Testosterone therapy has become a big part of our treatment protocol because of its safety and efficacy. The literature strongly supports its use, however, as discussed above, the FDA and endocrine societies do not. I find this very unfortunate because of the potential benefit in so many spheres of healthspan! For bone mineral density (BMD) and muscle mass specifically, consider the following:

- A 2004 randomized controlled trial on 33 premenopausal women treated with topical testosterone demonstrated an increase in bone turnover markers in an at-risk population (Miller, 2004).
- A 2011 prospective cohort study on 61 postmenopausal women treated with estradiol and testosterone pellets showed improved bone mineral density after 12 months of almost 2% in spine and 4% in the hips! More than would be expected from estrogen therapy alone (Britto, 2011).
- A 2008 prospective, randomized, single-blinded trial on 34 women compared either estrogen and progestin alone or in combination with testosterone and showed that both groups improved BMD, but the addition of testosterone demonstrated superior improvements in BMD again than estradiol alone or in combination with progestins (Davis, 2008).
- A 2023 meta-analysis looking at men showed increases in both bone density and lean muscle mass (Buratto, 2023). Unfortunately, studies evaluating lean muscle mass gains in

women have not been done, so we can't clearly identify what the gains would be in our population of interest.

We also have reviewed numerous additional studies on men demonstrating the benefits of testosterone therapy alone on BMD. It is clear that the anabolic impact of testosterone will improve bone density with or without estrogen, but the bias in this research is clearly toward men. This realization becomes very important when having a conversation around HRT with women who may not be candidates for estrogen therapy, although there are likely less women in that category than most think! More on that in future chapters. Many practitioners view HRT as a singular tool with one recommended form and dose. I strongly disagree. HRT is not an all-or-nothing phenomenon and not a one-size-fits-all tool to consider. Testosterone, specifically, can be used independently of estradiol and provide tremendous benefits, but as discussed previously, is "off label" according to the FDA for, well, everything!

Some patients are afraid to start testosterone because of concerns around negative mood changes with use. There is a misconception that testosterone can result in aggressive behavior. Not only is this not seen in the literature, but actually testosterone often shows improvement in mental health. Psychological well-being is actually quite difficult to measure, particularly in high-functioning individuals. True clinical depression is often obvious, but a depressed mood and subtle changes that can be very impactful may not be so easily identified. I see this in patients who would not be classified as depressed clinically but after starting testosterone therapy report improvement in depressed feelings. I personally felt this shift when optimizing my own hormones. The literature supports this as well. A 2003 randomized controlled trial on 34 premenopausal women with the average age of 40 used testosterone cream for 3 months and used an index of psychological general well-being, a sexual self-rating scale and a depression inventory score to measure outcomes. The testosterone therapy improved all three but less so with the depression score. This is not surprising since the participants were not required to be depressed as an inclusion criteria for the study. I wouldn't expect to improve something that isn't present (Goldstat, 2003). However, a study that intentionally included depressed patients did indeed show improved symptoms when depression was a clear starting point (Miller, 2004). So testosterone alone seems to at a minimum improve psychological well-being and depression when present. Aggression was not noted in any participant.

I was disappointed to read that the American College of Obstetricians and Gynecologists (ACOG) published a statement raising a red flag around testosterone use and breast cancer. They specifically note that an association between testosterone and breast cancer has been reported. Indeed, there are studies that notice generally nonsignificant increases in short-term studies from 6–12 months in length. Let's explore this finding and other studies that will likely help you feel at ease with testosterone therapy and the risk of breast cancer.

First, let's explore some statistics around breast cancer. Sadly, it's common and becoming more common. Statistically, 1 in 8 women will be diagnosed with breast cancer in her lifetime. This makes breast cancer the most common cancer diagnosis in women. It's not surprising then that studies performed on women at risk for this cancer will turn up cases of cancer. However, as we have discussed in the "Reason #2" chapter on estrogen, the genesis and timeline associated with breast cancers needs to be considered with certain study designs. For cancers to be identified on imaging studies like mammograms, they have to reach at least a few millimeters in size. While still small, these cancers contain millions of cancer cells and generally will take many months if not years to develop. Consider then if a 6-month study shows an increase in breast cancer incidence or diagnosis. Did the intervention cause it, or was it there before the study started but not large enough to identify on imaging studies? Likely the latter. That's why we need more than one study and consistency in findings to be sure that what we are seeing is truly an increase and not a random increase by chance.

Fortunately, there are multiple studies which can help us feel certain of the safety of testosterone in this regard. When compared to the expected rates of breast cancer incidence, a 2019 study of over 1,200 participants using testosterone pellets demonstrated that the rates of breast cancer detection in the testosterone group was lower than would be expected for a control group not on testosterone therapy by 40%! That's a big difference (Glaser, 2019). This appears to be due to testosterone's ability to impact the breast on a cellular level. In a 2007 randomized controlled trial, 99 participants on an estradiol/progestin HRT product were given either testosterone or placebo (Hofling, 2007). After 6 months, the participants were subjected to a biopsy of breast tissue and the numbers of proliferating breast cells compared between groups. This is relevant because proliferation of breast cells can lead to an increased risk of cancer. The placebo group had a five-fold increase in cell proliferation compared to the testosterone group! They concluded that testosterone therapy likely counteracted breast cell proliferation induced by estrogen and progestin therapy in postmenopausal women. In other words, testosterone may be protective of breast cancer. This was echoed by a 2009 review paper looking at both human and primate studies (Dimitrakakis, 2009).

While this may be surprising in some ways, it shouldn't be really. As mentioned above, testosterone is a major player in the symphony of hormones in a woman's body. Why would it be surprising that testosterone may play a role in balancing estrogen and progesterone? The biggest question remaining for me when considering testosterone is the other potential risks outside of breast cancer. We've discussed some of the well-known potential side effects in the studies already, but there are some larger studies looking to prove safety exclusively, which can give us even more insight.

A 2009 study looking at a large database in the UK, looking at over 2,100 women using testosterone and over 6,300 controls, compared the rates of complications, like stroke, heart disease, breast cancer, blood clots, diabetes and liver inflammation. There was no increase in the testosterone group (Van Staa, 2009). A 2019 meta-analysis of 46 reports and 36 randomized controlled trials on 8,480 participants brought up concerns of increased levels of LDL cholesterol which some studies report (Islam, 2019). This type of evidence is often cited with concerns of an increased risk of heart disease and events with testosterone and androgens. There are two issues with this assumption. First, it assumes that increasing

LDL cholesterol is associated with increased heart disease, which it can be but is not always. Particularly in women, metabolic health is a much more important risk factor than LDL cholesterol, but we can't say for certain that these women were metabolically healthy. Interestingly, there is at least one study that also demonstrated potentially worsening metabolic health as measured through insulin resistance with testosterone (Zang, 2006). If worsening metabolic health and increasing LDL cholesterol were consistently seen with testosterone use, that would indeed be a problem. Fortunately, both of these risks were only seen with oral administration of testosterone, not topical.

Testosterone is highly metabolized by the liver and creates undesirable metabolic byproducts with undesirable effects. I don't recommend oral administration of testosterone due to these and other liver issues seen with historically tested products. While large intervention trials focusing specifically on heart disease and testosterone in women have not been done, we can look at the recent 2023 RCT performed on men to help us clarify the confusion here. The TRAVERSE trial was a multicenter, randomized, double-blind, placebo-controlled trial on 5,246 men aged 45–80 who were considered high risk for cardiovascular disease and were truly "hypogonadal" with total testosterone levels below 300 ng/dL. The average treatment with a testosterone gel was a little under two years with follow-up data out to almost 3 years.

Analysis of these data revealed less "cardiovascular primary endpoints," which in this study specifically was a fatal or nonfatal heart attack or stroke. While this study was applauded as a large trial that supports testosterone replacement in men that need it, I wish it were longer in duration and that they used more physiologic doses of testosterone. I'm happy to see that there was no signal for increased risk, BUT I'd love to see the study continue for another 15–20 years. Unfortunately, funding for this duration and size of study on testosterone is not likely to be available, especially not in women! This is a scenario where we have to extrapolate the available data to women even though we don't want to treat women as small men. We have to use the available evidence rather than waiting for the ideal study to come along. In this case, it probably never will.

I go through the available literature on testosterone in this book not necessarily to make the case for testosterone replacement in all women. Remember that women CAN make 75% of their maximum testosterone production after menopause. There was a point in time when I felt like testosterone was the elixir of life. I used it myself. I recommended it frequently, and many of our patients saw benefits. However, there is a rarely discussed and not well-understood dark side to testosterone replacement that has encouraged me to look at alternatives in both my patients and my own health optimization.

We always want to look at hormone replacement through the lens of healthspan, meaning that we review additional biomarkers to look at overall health so we can verify that what we're doing is going to help us improve our healthspan. One of the areas that many of us suffer from is excess oxidative stress. We live in a stressful world, and oxidative stress parallels inflammation as two of the biggest drivers of disease. Part of the oxidative stress picture is iron metabolism and iron overload, especially in postmenopausal women. Cycling women have the ability to purge excess iron monthly through menses; postmenopausal women do not (unless on rhythmic HRT). Additionally, iron is a common element in our environment and has been erroneously added to many processed foods as a fortification to avoid deficiency. This is an issue because iron is very reactive and oxidative. Think of rust, the result of iron exposed to oxygen and water in our environment. Iron in our body goes through a similar process if not appropriately metabolized. Iron metabolism is a very complex topic that very few fully understand, including myself. But what has been made clear to me is that in some individuals, testosterone replacement increases iron absorption and can contribute to iron overload (Guo, 2013; Gabrielsen,

2017). I've seen this in myself and many patients. Excess oxidative stress will not help us live better or longer. And if testosterone increases biomarkers associated with oxidative stress and iron metabolism dysfunction, alternatives are worth considering.

Fortunately, there are dozens of studies on DHEA for androgen replacement, but the results are mixed. Why? Because when we switch to less powerful over-the-counter (in the US) products, like DHEA, the host status is critical. DHEA will not make an impact on a sick body the way that testosterone may. Additionally, for clarity of outcomes, many of these studies used DHEA as an independent intervention and often at low doses that do not achieve adequate blood levels. In my experience, DHEA needs to be used in conjunction with optimized estradiol and progesterone AND a program to optimize adrenal function. Alone, this precursor is unlikely to be effective. One meta-analysis of RCTs came to this conclusion as well but interestingly did demonstrate that DHEA alone could reach significance for quality of life and depression but only trended that way for anxiety, libido and satisfaction with sex. Some of the RCTs showed significant improvement and some did not (Alkatib, 2009).

So, what's the answer? Androgens are important for women IF NEEDED. However, testosterone is NOT a panacea and is not required by all or probably most women if estradiol and progesterone are optimized. But Reason #5 why your hormone replacement is failing you may simply be that you need more androgens! What to use and in combination with what else are points of nuance that require an adequate lab, history and symptom review.

REASON #6

YOU'RE "TOO OLD" TO START HRT OR "TOO OLD" TO CONTINUE HRT (HEART AND BRAIN HEALTH)

To have a discussion with your doctor around the risks and benefits of HRT, both you and your doctor need to understand both sides of the equation. Your doctor is not likely to have a good understanding of the updated risks and benefits, so it's imperative that you do.

We've discussed in the studies presented so far that the risk of cancer and heart disease seems minimal if we eliminate synthetic progestins from the mix. Now let's discuss the benefit side of the equation when it comes to heart (and brain) health. Research in this area is challenging, both to do and to interpret. There are many studies and many forms of HRT, which can be confusing, but with a clear route through the trees, I think we can see the forest.

Estrogen is without a doubt a factor in heart and vascular health. There are numerous mechanisms in which estrogen is thought to maintain or potentially improve heart health with replacement. However, the studies on this topic present confusing and contradictory data. The biggest areas of discussion are: when to start, when to stop and what to do if you already fall outside of these ideal parameters. This last point is challenging since we are now over 20 years after the first WHI publication and an entire generation of women have been impacted by the changes in HRT recommendations as well as the resistance to accept newer literature contradicting the studies from the early 2000's (even when from the same authors). Many women in this group are now in their 60's and early 70's and ask me often about whether or not they can start HRT. This is one of the more difficult discussions to have around HRT because these women in my practice also likely have osteoporosis and are desperately looking to avoid pharmaceutical management of their bone health. Fortunately, there are many slam dunk discussions to have around estrogen and heart health in different age populations. Let's start there and provide some context for our more difficult conversations with our older patients.

Estrogen has long been considered good for the heart and arteries. The hypothesis for heart health stems from observational studies demonstrating that women trail men in developing heart disease by about a decade. The onset of such disease generally coincides with the decade following menopause. The loss of estrogen during menopause was thought to bring women's risk more in line with men's. Multiple studies have been done to demonstrate the potentially beneficial impact of estrogen on arterial health. Estrogen has been shown to have a positive impact on cholesterol, which may play a role. But if you have heard me talk about cholesterol, you'll know that I don't believe that cholesterol is the primary risk factor to consider for heart disease. Other potential benefits of estrogen include anti-inflammatory and antioxidant effects, anti-platelet effects, improved arterial function and resistance to plaque formation (Naftolin, 2019). While this is a seemingly logical theory, there must be more to it because as I mentioned before, the WHI failed to show a heart health benefit in either the estrogen-only and combined HRT group, or at least initially. So, if estrogen is so good for the heart, why didn't this large trial show a benefit?

One of the interesting things about the WHI design is that it tried to compensate for the risk of participants knowing if they were on active HRT or placebo. The researchers were concerned that if women were overtly symptomatic in menopause with hot flashes and night sweats, they would know if they were on estrogen or not. To avoid this bias and likely high rate of dropout for those on placebo, they designed the trial to minimize the inclusion of women with symptoms of menopause. They report less than 10% of their participants had such symptoms. As a result of this criteria, they ended up with an older average population of postmenopausal women than would typically represent a group of symptomatic women. The average age in this study was 66 with the oldest being 78 years old. This group was clearly past 10 years from the onset of menopause, and therefore, represented a higher risk group for heart disease. It's not surprising then that their goal of identifying heart disease protection failed. This wasn't the right study group!

Fortunately, some researchers have evaluated the WHI data and stratified risk based on age and time since menopause. It's clear from these data that the earlier HRT is started after the onset of menopause or associated symptoms, the lower the potential risk, and in fact, there may be a favorable protective effect (Chester, 2018). In the 50–59 age group, women indeed saw a protective effect of estrogen for heart attack. The favorable impact was neutralized for the

60–69-year-old group, and there was a trend toward increased risk in the 70–79-year-old group. These data were only for the estrogen-alone group, NOT the combined-therapy group. The progestin likely increased risk as discussed previously. Additionally, two studies further exploring this topic were conducted and published to aid in this challenging discussion.

KEEPS is a study that was published in 2014 and evaluated 727 women within 3 years of menopause that had an average age of 52. They used oral or topical estradiol paired with micronized progesterone and evaluated progression of Carotid Intima Media Thickness (CIMT) and Coronary Artery Calcium (CAC) to establish changes in risk from the intervention versus placebo. There were no protective or deleterious effects from the 4-year trial on these measures (Harman, 2014). The Danish Osteoporosis Prevention Study looked at HRT and osteoporosis but also reported on the risk of heart disease in a younger group of women. This study not only showed no worsening of disease, but in fact, a statistically significant benefit from combined HRT for death, heart attack and heart failure with no increased risk of cancer, blood clot or stroke (Schierbeck, 2012). Lastly, long-term cohort studies, like the Nurses' Health Study (NHS), again show protection from heart attack in those within 4 years from menopause but also no increased risk regardless of the duration of hormone use (Bhupathiraju, 2016).

So, the data is pretty clear to me that starting HRT at the onset of menopause or symptoms associated with menopause is likely protective of vascular and heart health. This makes physiologic sense and is supported by the data. That's why we go out of our way to report on these studies and more through our social media and YouTube outlets. Women are not being informed of this benefit and the narrow window associated with it! Which leads me back to my patients in their 60s and 70s with osteoporosis and fear of fracture. To navigate the gray area here, we have a heart-to-heart with our patients about risk. In all of the studies I just mentioned, the increased risk is apparently real and gets larger as we get further away from menopause. The WHI data specifically points toward increased preexisting cardiovascular risk as the source of the difference between the younger women and the older. In other words, the increased risk of having a heart attack or stroke is due to the increases in risk factors that occur in the years following menopause. This time period is associated with increased risk of abnormal cholesterol, insulin resistance, obesity and oftentimes stress and inflammation. All of these can negatively impact heart health, and when they accumulate for years, the risk of having an event upon starting HRT seems to go up. However, not all of my patients do see these risk factors develop. Is it fair then to deny a healthy 65-year-old woman who is 11 years out from menopause HRT if she has not developed insulin resistance, high blood pressure, obesity, etc.? What if her arteries are clean as a whistle? Does her risk still go up? How do we know? This is where critical thinking and clinical decision making come into play.

We have the ability to stratify the risk of cardiovascular disease. Some of the studies use CIMT and CAC to define this risk and progression of disease, and these studies do provide value. In fact, we now perform a CAC on all patients over 50 that join our practice. However, CAC can have false negatives and provide false reassurance of absence of disease. The most compelling test available is the Coronary CT Angiogram (CCTA) with Cleerly. This is a CT like the CAC but tells us about narrowing of the arteries as well as soft plaque in addition to the calcified plaque. The CCTA is done in a hospital imaging suite, while the Cleerly is performed as a software add-on behind the scenes by my team. When patients are willing to perform this test, it gives us great insight into disease progression and possible risk. I recently reviewed two studies on women in their late 60s with osteoporosis desperate to start on HRT who had absolutely no plaque buildup in their coronary arteries. Should I deny them HRT based on risk that doesn't seem to apply to them? No, I started them on HRT, and they are doing very well.

All of the papers I reviewed that demonstrate potential benefit for women from HRT regarding heart health echo the concerns of the WHI and state in one way or another that HRT should not be used as a preventive measure for heart disease. I understand that by recommending to do so would raise red flags and put the authors at risk of being in the crosshairs of the pharmaceutical industry, American Heart Association and more, but what then should we call it? When I have a patient that is 52, within 4 years from menopause, symptomatic, osteopenic and concerned about heart disease, do I tell her that we only give her HRT for her symptoms of menopause? Are we not also protecting her bones and her heart? Is it unethical as a physician to suggest that she is likely to see cardioprotection from the HRT? Perhaps I just don't say anything; after all, she does have symptoms of menopause, so I can write that into her chart and move on. That doesn't jive with my integrity as a physician or researcher. I believe that we should disclose the potential benefits as well as risk! Let's say this same 52-year-old doesn't have symptoms of menopause, isn't osteopenic but is only worried about heart disease prevention. What do I do now? Refuse her HRT because the studies say not to use it for heart disease prevention? Ask her another way if she has symptoms of menopause so I can justifiably write that into her medical record? These are some of the tricky situations physicians face every day around HRT! It feels like dancing around land mines and helps explain why many physicians want nothing to do with it.

Lastly, what about dementia? This is another area of controversy but without as much evidence supporting either side of the argument. There is conflicting data around dementia and HRT. What makes this area more difficult to study than heart disease is that the brain is harder to access and leaves us fewer clues. The blood brain barrier makes biomarkers less useful at unwrapping the mysteries of the brain, but some data is available to review. Again, if we look at the WHI data for which we have over 20 years of data, we can see some compelling results. In an 18-year follow-up publication on mortality in the HRT vs placebo groups, the researcher reported a significant reduction in death from dementia in those using oral estradiol alone compared to placebo or progestins (Manson, 2017). However, studies such as the 2019 Finnish cohort study showed a subtle increased risk of dementia with exposure (Savolainen-Peltonen, 2019). A newer meta-analysis published in 2023 may help to shed light on this issue. When observational studies and randomized controlled trials are compared together, what these authors found is that when HRT is started within 10 years of menopause estrogen therapy, in particular, it appears to be protective of dementia. After 10 years, the benefit is less clear. Additional findings in this study point toward less protection with synthetic progestins and potential harm (Nerattini, 2023). Most recently, an analysis of HRT use after the age of 65 was published which demonstrated that those with continued use of estrogen after the age of 65 were protected from dementia (Baik, 2024).

The mechanism in which estrogen may be neuroprotective is robust. We've already discussed how the vascular effect can improve cardiovascular risk. Some forms of dementia are very clearly vascular based, but vascular health may indirectly play a role in other forms of dementia. Additionally, estrogen is anti-inflammatory, which should be protective of dementia as well. Estrogen has also been implicated in amyloid metabolism, which is thought to be a driver of Alzheimer's specifically as well as neuroplasticity, which can impact our ability to compensate for changes as we age. The potential benefits are long, but the large studies shouldn't be ignored. When it comes to recommendations though, I feel similarly thwarted by the general consensus which seems to be that estrogen should not be used for dementia prevention. I agree that the evidence isn't clear, but I find it interesting when a woman goes through an early menopause for whatever reason that estrogen is often recommended to prevent the onset of hormone-related cognitive decline, but when estrogen withdrawal occurs naturally, the same recommendations are not made. Why would we treat a 40-year-old so differently than a 50-year-old? This is where viewing hormone replacement through the lens of healthspan can be so critically important. More on that later.

So, Reason #6 that your hormone replacement isn't working is that someone told you not to start or to stop because of heart or brain health when that may not have been in your best interest. Many doctors want to discontinue use of HRT after 10 years or after the age of 65. From a longevity perspective, this is absolutely illogical unless the risk/benefit equation changed due to another diagnosis. Sadly, longevity studies in humans are notoriously difficult to do. Fortunately, a recent study mentioned above looking at women continuing on HRT after the age of 65 showed remarkable benefits! In this study, continued estrogen replacement was associated with significant reductions in:

- Mortality (19%)
- Breast Cancer (16%)
- Lung Cancer (13%)
- Colon Cancer (12%)
- Heart Attack (11%)

Combined therapy did not fare as well, in my opinion, due to the nature of systemic progestin therapy. I often get a sense that HRT is put in a position of guilty until proven innocent, and this is a great example. From a longevity perspective, why would continued hormones at low or even physiologic levels be dangerous? Shouldn't we be looking for evidence of harm and proving that hypothesis rather than assuming it causes harm and proving it doesn't? From my perspective trying to help people live better, longer, this is the angle we take, which brings me to another contentious topic. Physiologic HRT. Physiologic HRT can mean two things from my perspective: physiologic levels and rhythmic dosing. We'll start with physiologic levels.

REASON #7

MAYBE YOU SIMPLY NEED MORE?

Research around optimal estradiol levels for specific goals in postmenopausal women is lacking, but the quest for optimal health pushed me to explore what evidence does exist. This was extremely relevant for the development of our osteoporosis program where we consistently saw patients coming into our program on low dose HRT that were still losing bone. These women were shocked to learn that the estrogen that they were taking to support their bone health was not protecting their bone. Their HRT was "failing them."

We shouldn't blame the estradiol though. It didn't fail them. What I've found is some compelling evidence to support the idea that certain tissues are going to respond to estradiol at different serum levels. In addition to that, there is likely variation from person to person in the levels necessary to see the results we are aiming for.

Unfortunately, we don't have the evidence I want to see available to us. What I want to see is a trial looking at different levels of estradiol with replacement and measuring outcomes related to estrogen deficiency as we've previously described. That study has never been done to my knowledge, but we do have compelling evidence to review. It's mostly around bone health because bones are easier to measure than other outcomes, like mood, cognitive function and cardiovascular health. Bone metabolism leaves a trail to follow, and that can help guide our dosing to some degree.

In a review of the SWAN bone study, the authors identified that as women transitioned into menopause, the average levels of estradiol were strongly associated with bone mineral density and that the threshold of 35 pg/mL was the tipping point (Lo, 2011). That may be attainable with low dose HRT, but two additional studies on postmenopausal women showed a range of 70–90 pg/mL of estradiol were required to maintain bone (Reginster, 1992; Zhu, 2021). This level of estrogen is pushing what we can safely provide in a static manner due to what's known as the physiologic ceiling of static HRT.

We can only provide so much progesterone orally without achieving a sedating side effect, and as a result, we can only provide so much estradiol before we create an imbalance in the endometrial lining of the uterus. More of both at the same time may not provide the benefits we are looking for anyway. The physiology of the human body can only tolerate so much of both hormones at one time without either provoking breakthrough bleeding or putting a woman at risk for endometrial cancer or both. The question then should be, "Is that okay? Can we use these hormones at static doses and achieve our goals? Maybe, but consider the evidence for improved outcomes with more physiologic doses." We know that the amount of estradiol to reduce or eliminate hot flashes is much lower than levels known to impact bone. As mentioned above, there are multiple studies indicating that levels from 60–80 pg/mL in serum may be an inflection point for bone turnover markers and associations with osteoporosis (Huitron-Bravo, 2016; Zhu, 2021; Hadji, 2019; Reginster, 1992). This level coincides with the average estradiol level at the end of the early follicular phase. However, this level of estrogen is quite low compared to the late follicular phase and even the luteal phase of the menstrual cycle. It is a little over half of the statistical average estradiol level if you were to average the entire month for the "average" woman. Using the average levels may be logical but likely crosses the physiologic ceiling of estradiol that we can use due to the limitations in progesterone dosing orally. There is actually one study that showed the difference between low and higher dose estradiol on bone. They used three different doses of topical estradiol and the highest dose performed the best. In my opinion this isn't surprising! (Yang, 2007) The study with the highest serum estradiol levels I found hit around 90pg/mL in a rhythmic manner with topical patches. Interestingly, they compared these results to a much higher dose of static estradiol and estriol reaching serum estradiol levels of over 230 pg/mL but the lower dose group out performed the higher dose group. Why? It likely had to do with the timing. More on that later. (Stanosz, 2009)

Even if we stay within the known boundaries of static dosing, we can likely achieve serum levels identified to improve bone health. While that's great for those looking to improve bone health, what about levels required for other tissues? I'd love to know what levels we need for optimal vascular, cardiac and brain health. Even with what we know for bone health, my fear is that these levels are inflection points of bone loss, but are they adequate for bone building? Sadly, the fear of estrogen has deterred research looking at nuance like estradiol levels for various tissues. This is why when I treat patients, we do so through the lens of healthspan and measure biomarkers that help us differentiate the function of these and other organs to the best of our ability.

Each woman's ability to tolerate "higher" levels of static HRT is likely going to vary greatly from person to person. Regardless of how high we push these levels, we will fail to achieve true physiologic levels. On average, women see spikes of estradiol to 250 pg/mL in the late follicular phase and around 130 pg/mL in the luteal phase with remarkable variation. Could it be that we need to achieve these levels to truly see the maximal benefits of HRT? Reason #7 your hormones aren't working for you? You simply don't have enough to achieve the goals you are looking for.

Progesterone dosing and testosterone dosing are entirely different rabbit holes to consider. Physiologic testosterone levels are not difficult to obtain, but clinical responses tend to be variable. Progesterone levels are challenging to measure when using oral therapy and impossible to measure in venous blood when using topical preparations. So then, maybe we need to continue to cycle hormones in replacement like women do naturally before menopause. Stick with me here as we go down this rabbit hole. You may just find what you're looking for on the other side.

REASON #8

MAYBE YOU NEED TO MENSTRUATE?

As an outsider looking at traditional HRT for women, I have to admit that the entire principle and approach seems flawed. If we want to optimize hormone function, why would we take two hormones (estrogen and progesterone), which used to have an obvious monthly alternating rhythm, and then "replace" them in a static (same daily dose) manner?

BioIdentical HRT refers to compounds that are biologically identical to those endogenously produced BUT not at bioidentical levels or rhythmically as they were produced before menopause. It seems intuitive then that if we truly wanted to optimize hormones after menopause, we would mimic the compounds (bioidentical), physiologic doses and cyclic rhythm of estrogen and progesterone through physiologic restoration (PR).

I'd like to be up front and honest with you about where I am in the evolution of this approach in my practice. I'm interested in the potential benefit, BUT with limited evidence with this style of prescribing, we are left to read between the lines of the available literature to establish safety and possible benefits. I currently have a team of just under 30 employees. They are nearly all women. The first time I brought up this topic to my team, I felt "a bit" of resistance. However, after describing the potential benefits, I had a Zoom screen of nodding heads. The most common question we get is around menstruation, and if you are scratching your head right now and wondering if rhythmic, physiologic replacement will cause a monthly bleed in women with a uterus, the answer is, yes. While this may be appalling to many women, I have spoken to both providers and patients using physiologic restoration who are more than happy to experience the "inconvenience" of a monthly bleed for the benefits they have experienced. One of my passions in medicine is to uncover controversial discrepancies and expose the potential benefits of hidden treatments. This is certainly one of those areas. I don't think this will replace our traditional static HRT dosing anytime soon, but let me walk you through the compelling evidence that may point toward physiologic restoration as an option for those that aren't seeing the benefits they would expect from a traditional static approach.

My first introduction to this concept was during a review of the Danish study that showed a protection from heart attack in "cyclic combined" therapy, which was in contrast to a significant increase in heart attack risk in continuous or static combined therapy. Initially, I missed this all together, but later I recognized that they were talking about cycling progesterone. One of the challenges of this study is that there are many ways to cycle progesterone and they did not break down these subgroups, but further investigation continues to support physiologic benefits of progesterone withdrawal which mimicks the end of the luteal phase of the menstrual cycle (Lokkegaard, 2008). Remember that these hormones have receptors everywhere and their actions are unique to one another. What if the presence or absence of these hormones was not coincidental but required for the optimal function of estradiol and progesterone? I want to run through all of the potential benefits but let's first explore bone health as an example of a tissue that clearly responds to cycling hormones.

Estradiol is known to have a big impact on bone health, and fortunately, bone metabolism leaves a trail of biomarkers to follow, which do improve with enough estradiol. That's why I use it whenever possible in our bone health programs. There are multiple mechanisms at play here, but a big one is the inhibition of osteoclast differentiation, which slows bone loss. This is most apparent naturally at the highest levels of estradiol in the late follicular phase. As estradiol levels fall from its peak around day 12, bone loss accelerates and makes room for bone development by osteoblasts. The rise of progesterone in the luteal phase promotes bone formation. While each hormone plays a role, it's the alternating surges that allow for natural bone metabolism. I was shocked when I revisited evidence on bone health trials in the 90's and early 2000's that most of the studies were using some form of rhythmic dosing! What is even more compelling about these studies is that some of them compare static dosing to rhythmic dosing and the results were always superior when hormones were cycled. This was true even when the blood levels of estradiol in the static group was 2.5X higher than in the rhythmic group! (Gonnelli, 1997, Adami, 1989, Yang 2007, Stanosz, 2009, Hosking, 1998, Ettinger, 2004)

There is even evidence to support the idea that a certain number of cycles per year is required for optimal bone development and health. A 2010 review identified that women need to have at least 5 "normal" cycles per year to maintain bone and that progesterone at physiologic levels is required for optimal bone formation through the progesterone pathway (Seifert-Klauss, 2010). In our bone health program, we currently use oral micronized progesterone and topical estradiol in a static fashion, meaning we do not cycle or change doses of either hormone during the month. We do see improvements in bone biomarkers in our patients with this protocol, however, these data and the future points in this chapter have been compelling enough to update our protocols and offer additional options for our patients.

When I discuss physiologic HRT with both patients and team members, the first question that everyone has is "What about breast cancer risk?" I find this fascinating since my patients and my team have listened to me dispute the dogma around estrogen and breast cancer time and time again. As stated in previous chapters, the evidence that estradiol causes breast cancer does not exist. There is no evidence for causation, only association. Additionally, in long follow-up studies, estrogen is protective of breast cancer. Physiologically, this has always made sense. If estrogen was truly causative of breast cancer, wouldn't we see the abundance of these cancers when women have more estrogen, before menopause? We should also see a decline of breast cancer after menopause in women who are not on replacement. Neither of those scenarios are true, so why do we assume that more estrogen would cause an increased risk of breast cancer?

Fortunately, when it comes to breast tissue, we do have some data to help guide us. First, there is evidence to support the idea that breast tissue absolutely changes based on the levels of each hormone during the menstrual cycle. The ratio of estradiol to progesterone appears to have a visible impact on the glandular tissue of the breast. I think this is intuitive to most women but has been debated in the medical literature. Surgical specimens correlated to reported cycle phase and serum hormone levels confirm that the tissue does indeed change throughout the cycle (Ramakrishnan, 2002). These tissue changes also appear to be associated with changes in genomic expression. The tumor suppressor genes, TOB1 and p53 as well as Bcl-2, involved in cell apoptosis are all upregulated with progesterone at physiologic levels (Formby, 1998; Azeez, 2015). Clinically, this plays out with a 5x increase in breast cancers in premenopausal women with a progesterone deficiency that limits the effect of progesterone on cell apoptosis and tumor suppression (Cowan, 1981).

There is also evidence that surgery for breast cancer has better disease-free and survival outcomes when performed during the luteal as opposed to the follicular phase of the menstrual cycle (Jatoi, 1998).

The elevated levels of progesterone with functional receptors suppresses tumor formation and promotes apoptosis of old cells. I agree that a trial with physiologic dosing and progesterone cycling would help me to feel better about the recommendation I'm suggesting, but like most things in the health optimization space, we need to consider the data that's available to help us make a risk:benefit analysis. Breast health seems to be favored with progesterone cycling.

Cardiovascular health also appears to be impacted by the cycling of sex hormones in women. Women have lower rates of cardiovascular disease than men before menopause. Higher levels of estrogen are often credited for this health benefit, but the mechanisms are not clearly understood. One hypothesis is the increased number of endothelial progenitor cells in women when they cycle naturally. Endothelial progenitor cells (EPCs) are formed in the bone marrow and can be identified in blood. They provide numerous benefits to the vascular system, including formation and repair of blood vessels, promoting a healthy artery lining (endothelium) and reducing plaque formation in the arteries (atherosclerosis). EPC volume is remarkably different between men and women, with higher levels found in women. Estradiol plays a critical role in the development of EPCs, and as it turns out, EPC levels are at their highest during the follicular phase of the menstrual cycle when estrogen levels are at their highest. After menopause, EPC levels decline to those of age-matched men. Again, supporting the idea that surging levels of estrogen alternating with progesterone serve a purpose beyond generating menstruation and that low-dose static HRT is likely not adequate to reproduce these same benefits, and remember that heart disease (not breast cancer) is the number one killer of women over the age of 65 (Fadini, 2008).

Another area for possible HRT improvement is seen at the cellular level. Estrogen and progesterone play an integral role in each other's ability to function as a hormone. Hormones are only one side of the communication pathway in the body. They are outgoing messages. Receiving tissues need receptors to understand the communication signal coming through the hormones. Receptor density and dysfunction are possible reasons for HRT failure. From a receptor perspective, estradiol plays a role in increasing both progesterone and estradiol receptors in tissues. Progesterone plays the counterpart of reducing expression of these same receptors. When static dosing is utilized, the estradiol and progesterone signaling for receptors is constantly contradictory, which may result in dysfunction and failure to achieve our HRT goals. Receptor function and density is difficult to study, but this hypothesis could play out in a randomized trial looking at health outcomes.

Lastly, when we compare women's HRT to that of men's TRT, we see stark contrast in the goals and type of care. The goal of testosterone replacement for men is not to provide the lowest amount possible to relieve some of the symptoms but to provide an adequate amount of testosterone to relieve the symptoms of deficient testosterone. To achieve this goal, we will frequently replenish a man's testosterone level to that of his younger self when he looked and felt his best. I'm also a fan of physiologic daily dosing of testosterone in men to mimic the natural rhythm of testosterone production. I do this respecting possible side effects and monitoring blood levels of specific biomarkers, but I don't worry about increasing risk with increasing dose. In fact, because of the physiologic levels, I see less side effects when dosed this way. Why would we expect women to be different in this regard? Shouldn't restoring physiologic levels be the goal and changes made based on RCT evidence? We got to where we are now because the commercial products available early in the development of HRT could not mimic the physiologic levels of hormones, so the research was done on synthetic static dosing. You could argue that we are considering the wrong baseline and again looking at physiologic levels as "guilty until proven innocent." In my training there was no discussion of rhythmic dosing. Yet, when I review the literature for bone health in particular there are numerous studies showing the benefit and some current published recommendations still state that progesterone should be given cyclically. So, what happened? Well, in the post WHI era two things occurred. First, the concept of "as low as possible for as short a time as possible" became the default. While we know that's no longer necessary this concept squashed nearly all rhythmic dosing that used increasing and decreases doses of estradiol. Secondly, there was a big push for providers to recognize breakthrough bleeding as pathologic. This awareness campaign likely helped identify possible uterine cancers BUT also cast doubt on any protocols that provoked breakthrough bleeding or an actual menstrual cycle.

While there are no large trials looking only at physiologic restoration compared to static for multiple health outcomes there are reasonably sized trials using rhythmic protocols in the bone health space. A 1998 trial for the drug Fosamax enrolled over 1,600 women with half using rhythmic dosing and half static. In case you were wondering, the rhythmic group far outperformed the static group from a bone health perspective. (Hoskings, 1998) With this and numerous smaller trials in hand we can reassure our patients that these principles are not new and untested. They have not been tested with the same rigor as a trial such as the WHI would test them but there is interest. The NIH recently approved funding for one such study. Further evidence is in the works to demonstrate that we may be missing out on the optimal benefit of hormone therapy by sticking to the relatively new static dosing model.

I see so many patients that have not done well on static low-dose HRT and hear thousands of additional stories through our YouTube and social media outlets. Could it be that this is a solution for at least some of them? I don't think all women will want to continue to experience monthly menstruation for the remainder of their life, but as evidence continues to climb and more and more physicians get behind the idea, we may see the movement regain momentum. Reason #8 your hormones are failing you is that to achieve your goals, you may need to continue to cycle as you did before menopause.

REASON #9

YOU'RE STRUGGLING TO PUT IT ALL TOGETHER!

So, how do we move forward? We have clearly demonstrated that HRT is a powerful tool in the battle for health optimization. It has the power to relieve the symptoms that come along with menopause and aging that include the usual hot flashes and night sweats but also so much more. We can see improvement in energy, vitality, strength, body composition, sleep, performance, mood and the list goes on and on.

We can prevent bone loss and even improve bone health, delay or even reverse cardiovascular risk and possibly do the same for dementia. A logical discussion with the risks and benefits of HRT and how they relate to you specifically is a must, but this conversation MUST be had with a provider who truly understands the current evidence exposing the updated risks of HRT! The risks as I've described them are based on current evidence, not the risks as they were passed on through dogma or outdated medical society guidelines from the Endocrine Society, North American Menopause Society or The American College of Obstetricians and Gynecologists.

You have to find a provider who has done the research themselves and is comfortable putting together your unique risks and benefits. Once the decision has been made to move forward, the next question is how? How do we provide HRT with the most benefit and least risk? How do we help you optimize your hormones? Clearly, this book can't provide specific medical advice, but let me show you how we put this together in general.

First, let's start with the most controversial hormone, estrogen. Nearly all of the available evidence is looking at estradiol. There is no compelling reason to consider any other estrogen metabolite. Based on the available evidence, estrogen should be given transdermally either through a compounded cream or a patch. The commercial products will come as a patch that is generally exchanged twice per week and comes in a few different dose options. Patches can work, but be careful as the commercial products are only designed to treat "typical" symptoms of menopause and are often not adequate to achieve desired systemic levels and cannot easily be used for rhythmic physiologic restoration. Remember that the amount of estradiol required to relieve hot flashes is much lower than the levels required to optimize bone health, and my suspicion is other targets, like heart and brain health, require higher doses as well.

That said, I have seen commercial patches provide adequate, and in some cases, too much estrogen for static dosing approaching and even surpassing the physiologic ceiling described earlier. That's why testing is critical here! We regularly test estradiol levels in blood to make sure we are seeing the levels we desire. While many doctors and societies will say otherwise, there is compelling evidence to support therapeutic blood levels for specific tissues. To protect the bones, heart and brain, we aim for a minimal therapeutic blood level of 60 pg/mL (Reginster, 1992).

Due to the limited dosing options and reported challenges with patches, compounded creams are my preferred route of estrogen replacement. It allows us to get away from the pharmaceutical industry altogether and use compounded pharmacies that are experts in making hormones. We recommend using 503b certified pharmacies instead of local 503a pharmacies to ensure quality and safety around the products produced. The 503b pharmacies produce these products on a large scale and use strict quality criteria and third-party testing to provide the highest quality product to both physicians and consumers. Creams are applied daily or sometimes twice daily and allow for subtle adjustments in dosing as a result. The topical route avoids the potential issues of oral dosing. Some evidence does support even oral estradiol as increasing the risk of blood clot, but we can simply avoid the argument altogether by using a topical route through either patch or cream. Injection of estradiol is also an option for those concerned about the impact of creams on children, partners and pets. This is not common, but as physiologic HRT becomes more accepted, I expect I will hear more requests for this route of estradiol.

Many readers of this book have likely used a commonly prescribed product in the functional and integrative medicine space called Bi-Est. Bi-Est is a combined product with estradiol and estriol, frequently with more of the latter. I'm not sure when this trend started, but I suspect it was done in an effort to "minimize" the risk of estradiol in the early post WHI period. I won't go into the research, but estriol is sometimes considered to be safer than estradiol. The problem with this clinically is that estriol isn't as potent an estrogen as estradiol, so the risk may go down but so does the benefit! We see this clearly in the bone health space. In a study comparing three different doses of estradiol the authors used estriol as a control because they knew that it wouldn't protect bone. Yes, you read that correctly. The authors used estriol alone because they knew these participants would continue to lose bone like someone not on HRT. That's exactly what happened. The estriol control group lost 1.44% of the BMD in 12 months the highest dose estradiol group gained 8.69%! (Yang, 2007) Estriol DOES NOT PROTECT BONE and likely not other tissues as well. We also don't have even a small fraction of the data on estriol that we do for estradiol, so safety isn't really well-established. Lastly, estriol is only present in the female body in significant quantities during pregnancy, so replacing supraphysiologic quantities with HRT doesn't make physiologic sense. I was trained to use Bi-Est but quickly switched in my practice to estradiol in an attempt to follow the best literature and up-to-date recommendations for my patients.

Bi-Est is an example of doctors making rational clinical decisions, but as the evidence changes, so should our practice of medicine. We simply don't have the evidence to support using estriol instead of estradiol. As an outsider and surgeon trained in intervention, I'm keenly aware that I am generally more accepting of risk than my medically trained counterparts. I understand as someone who used to perform big invasive surgeries that once I make an incision, I can't go back. I'm responsible for the outcome. While the same is true with prescribing hormones, I find that many medical providers try to pretend that what they are doing isn't the same as what they are afraid of. This avoidance of risk results in the practices of testosterone and estriol instead of estradiol, but remember that using a lesser studied approach to achieve the same results isn't necessarily reducing risk. That's an approach I could never consider as a surgeon, and I don't consider it now. If we need estradiol to do what we need to do, we should use estradiol if the *risk:benefit* ratio checks out and is thoroughly discussed with the patient.

In the traditional medical model, progesterone is only given to balance estrogen for women that maintain their uterus past menopause. As described above, this misses the opportunity to leverage progesterone receptors on many tissues in the body! We recommend progesterone to all women who meet our criteria for replacement whether they have a uterus or not. Why not leverage the impact on bones, arteries and the brain? Our preferred route at this time is oral because of the beneficial breakdown of oral progesterone to GABA receptor-stimulating compounds that can dramatically improve sleep. Why not stimulate receptors, balance estrogen and improve sleep all at the same time?

Topical progesterone cannot be measured in blood as it is circulated through the lymphatic tissue and capillary beds. To achieve truly physiologic levels though, we may need to use topical progesterone to avoid the previously mentioned physiologic ceiling of therapy. This should be done with caution in a woman with a uterus who is not participating in physiologic restoration. If using oral progesterone, commercial products are available in doses of 100 mg and 200 mg. This immediate-release product works for some women. However, I find that many women stop using HRT because they didn't tolerate the progesterone or felt they had side effects that may have come from the commercial progesterone. Unfortunately, commercial progesterone is made with suboptimal ingredients, such as peanut oil, lecithin, titanium dioxide, Yellow no. 10 and Red no. 40. To avoid these additives and realize additional benefits, we prefer to use a compounded product. This allows us the opportunity to compound more specific doses other than 100 mg and 200 mg. We find some women are very sensitive to progesterone and may need doses as low as 50 mg (generally not with a uterus) and up to 300 mg or more even for static dosing. Additionally, compounded progesterone can also be formulated in an extended-release formula, which may help with sleep and better balance the correct dose.

Dialing in progesterone can provide a massive improvement in symptoms of menopause and lifestyle. It should go without saying that synthetic progesterone (progestins) are NEVER recommended in my practice for any purpose whatsoever. This includes ALL birth control! These ARE NOT HRT, and in my opinion, should not be used as such.

Testosterone is the least used of these three hormones and the least understood. It is not typically included by traditional providers for all of the reasons mentioned above. Whether or not to use testosterone can be a challenging questions for both providers and patients. As I said, we use it frequently at OHH because we are treating patients who desperately need to build muscle and bone. Therefore, I am asking about and looking closely for symptoms of androgen deficiency in all of our patients. I also test and recommend testing for total and free testosterone levels to see what a starting point and therapeutic window looks like for our patients. If this isn't a part of your provider's practice and you are on HRT without testosterone, consider this one additional paper I'll put forward to you. In a 2009 review paper, the authors eloquently pointed out that while testosterone levels may be adequate in postmenopausal women, the application of HRT without testosterone will actually make testosterone levels worse. Some physicians believe that the application of estrogen will increase testosterone. But in both men and women, the feedback loop for testosterone production is based on estrogen, not testosterone. So, HRT with estradiol predictably will lower testosterone levels, making deficiency more likely (Dimitrakakis, 2009).

We, therefore, recommend replacing it with a topical cream or injection when necessary. Cream is preferred by most and can be applied once or twice daily. Injections are also an option for those that want to avoid the inconvenience of a cream OR are concerned about transference of the cream to children or partners. Injections are done either weekly or twice weekly and can be done subcutaneously or intramuscularly. Pellets are NOT recommended due to difficulties in dosing, higher levels and duration of side effects. Once pellets are in, they cannot be removed. If side effects occur, the patient is on a potentially terrible ride. This risk is unnecessary and generally only benefits the bottom line of the clinic where they are inserted.

The addition of supplements and thyroid replacement, while beyond this book's scope, are important considerations for complete health optimization. Supplements and additional hormones can play a significant role in some women's protocols. Effective thyroid management is crucial, and your provider should be able to test, diagnose, and treat thyroid health adequately. Unfortunately, the traditional system often falls short in the arena of thyroid and adequate direction with over-the-counter supplements. Reason #9 that your hormones aren't working for you? You don't have the support to put it all together in a logical and meaningful way!

REASON #10

YOU DON'T HAVE ACCESS!

Hormone replacement is a massive tool in health optimization, but as I pointed out above, there are endless treatment protocols with commercial, compounded and over-the-counter products.

When I hear comments about "HRT not working," I am saddened by the failure of these women's providers or the system as a whole. The "failure" could be from the wrong combination of hormones, inadequate dosing, excessive dosing, wrong route, lack of testosterone or more. These comments break my heart because these stories are often followed by a story of being dismissed by their prescribing physician and told that there is nothing else the doctor can do about it. I consider this medical gaslighting and irresponsible prescribing. Rather than throwing our hands in the air and giving up when the first attempt doesn't relieve symptoms, we should take a different approach. I see this play out in five distinct groups of women. Let's see where you fit in!

The most reliable group of women to benefit clinically from HRT are the women who have gone through menopause in the previous 10 years. In my opinion, ALL women in this group should have a thorough conversation of the risks and benefits of HRT regardless of the presence of vasomotor symptoms. Understanding natural testosterone levels in this group is critical as well. We can reliably guess that estrogen and progesterone levels are minimal, but testosterone production can continue at reasonable levels. Knowing if deficiency of testosterone is present could help in determining if certain symptoms may be the result of androgen deficiency or if looking elsewhere is indicated. This group is more likely to be able to find some form of HRT because the benefit profile is so profound, but low-dose static commercial options are the norm. This type of HRT is unlikely to truly optimize this patient population. If you are in this group and feeling "better," that's great, but how do you want to feel? What are your goals?

Postmenopausal women over 10 years out from menopause frequently knock on my virtual clinic door. Women in their 60s and 70s often were denied the conversation and potential benefits of HRT when they went through menopause. These women often struggle to find a provider who is willing to risk stratify their medical conditions with them. Understanding true cardiovascular risk versus statistical averages takes a thorough history and likely additional testing and imaging that most doctors are unwilling to do. We frequently help women in this group to risk stratify and start HRT if the benefits still outweigh the risks. As women in this group pass 20 years from menopause, the decision to start HRT gets harder. It can be done BUT is more rare. There may be alternative options in this group as well with off-label use of progesterone and/or testosterone without estrogen to help achieve goals.

Women with a history of breast cancer or strong family history of breast cancer are almost universally denied HRT. I understand the desire to prevent cancer and cancer recurrence. However, there is evidence to support using estrogen in this group of women. This is a challenging conversation that requires knowledge of the cancer history, grade, stage and receptor status. I respect a woman's right to choose her future and medical treatment options. I am willing to have this discussion and do prescribe in this situation under the right circumstances. This is an area of developing research, hope and sometimes heartbreaking decision making.

Premenopausal and perimenopausal women often feel there is nothing we can do to optimize their hormones. If they are still cycling, even irregularly, most doctors will not consider optimizing hormone levels. I agree that adding estrogen is usually not the first choice for these women, but because the adrenal glands play such a critical role in progesterone and testosterone production, we see women with hormonal imbalances that can easily be supported with off-label use of these hormones. Both progesterone or testosterone therapy can help women suffering from symptoms of estrogen dominance or testosterone deficiency respectively. Many women feel better with both. Having a discussion with a provider trained to identify the potential symptoms associated with testosterone and progesterone deficiencies with appropriate lab testing to verify blood levels of hormones is critical to hormone optimization in this population. For women still struggling with symptoms despite progesterone and testosterone optimization, physiologic and rhythmic estradiol can be helpful.

Lastly, we see women who are on some form of HRT frequently looking for optimized levels and further improvement in their dosing. They likely feel better but not how they want to feel on HRT. They have not met their goals of optimizing their energy, sleep, body composition, libido, sexual function and more. Many times, these women report that their providers don't believe in testing for hormone levels and refuse to modify their dose based on persistent symptoms. They are often on estradiol patches and commercial progesterone. The vast majority of these women are also not on testosterone. Some of these women have tried different forms of pellet therapy, oral birth control as HRT and over-the-counter options without success. If you are in this group, please hear me! There are numerous ways to optimize HRT! Understanding blood levels before and after therapy can help to dial in what you take and how you take it. I have never seen a patient not be able to tolerate a well-designed program that fits her specific needs. It all starts with blood work and a consultation. Reason #10 that your hormones aren't working for you? You don't have access. We can fix that.

PART 3

THE PATH FORWARD

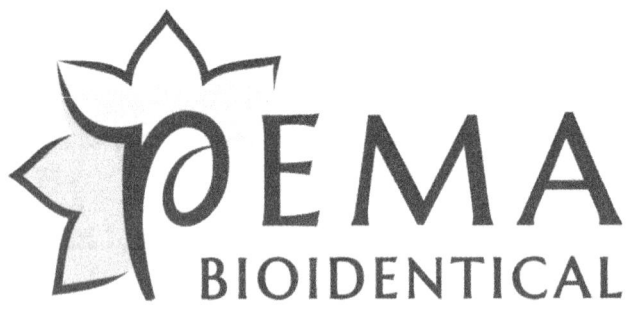

INTRODUCING PEMA BIOIDENTICAL

This book is not meant to be an advertisement. It is designed to be an easy-to-read guide for you to find some truth in the confusion around HRT and understand why your HRT may not be working the way you want it to. However, I think it would be unfair to show you the treasure that optimized hormones is but not offer you a path to get there. Consider one of the fruits of the last decade of my medical career, PEMA BioIdentical. If you have everything you need, I wish you well on your journey. If you need more support, aren't feeling as good as you want to or simply want to learn about your options, read on.

I never dreamed that I would spearhead a hormone replacement company for women. However, I have accepted that my mission in life is to educate and guide my patients toward optimal health. My overarching "Why" to life is to pursue Freedom and Love. My Why drives my How, and that is my mission. My mission to educate must go beyond the boundaries of OHH. Keeping this knowledge and opportunity to myself, my team and our patients at OHH does not fulfill my bigger purpose. Our program at OHH does incredible work for hundreds of patients, but not everyone wants or needs that level of care. For those that are simply in need of BHRT and thyroid replacement done how we do it at a reasonable price, we launched PEMA BioIdentical. PEMA, which means lotus in Tibetan, is needed because patients can't get what they know they need from their traditional practitioners or elsewhere in the chaos that is our medical system. PEMA BioIdentical was built to offer a streamlined virtual process to get you the testing, consultation and follow-up you need to get you feeling your best through hormone optimization. It all starts with a simple blood test. Visit us at: www.pemabioidentical.com for more on how to get started.

WHO IS DR. DOUG?

Dr. Doug Lucas is a double board-certified physician and founder of PEMA BioIdentical and Optimal HumanHealth MD (OHH), his two parallel platforms created with patient expectations and outcomes in mind. As a pioneer in the fields of healthspan, hormone replacement, osteoporosis and comprehensive telehealth solutions, Dr. Doug launched his nationwide telehealth practice to see patients in 2020. He created a platform that allowed him and his hand-picked team of experts to see patients the way they feel patients deserve to be seen.

Prior to Optimal Human Health MD, Dr. Doug practiced in the traditional medical model. He completed his orthopedic surgery training at Stanford University and began traditional orthopedic surgery practice in Durango, CO. After seven years of disappointment with the system in which Dr. Doug found himself, he left the traditional medical model and pursued additional training. He completed a fellowship with the American Academy of Anti-Aging Medicine (A4M) in anti-aging, hormone optimization, metabolic and functional medicine as well as a separate fellowship in epigenetics. After completion of this training, Dr Doug achieved his second Board Certification in Anti-Aging and Regenerative Medicine as well as the status of Fellow in Anti-Aging and Metabolic Medicine before fulfilling his vision by launching Optimal Human Health MD (OHH).

Shortly after launching the core program for healthspan with OHH and treating patients with the Health Optimization Pyramid framework, Dr. Doug used this backbone to create the "4R Method" to Recognize, Reverse, Retest and Revive patients with osteoporosis and osteopenia. OHHMD is now focused exclusively on bone health and stands alone as the only program run by a dual board-certified physician and surgeon with a team of experts to help patients get to the root problem of their bone loss, improve their healthspan and live without the fear of fracture.

During the rapid growth of OHH, Dr. Doug was exposed to the current state of hormone replacement in the US and worldwide. He and his team realized the tremendous need for a new approach to HRT that can be delivered through a telehealth platform and straight to a patient's door. This need drove Dr. Doug to found his second company, PEMA BioIdentical.

Dr. Doug maintains his memberships to the American Academy of Anti-Aging Medicine (A4M), the International Peptide Society (IPS) and the American Osteopathic Academy of Orthopedics (AOAO). He served on the research committee for the American Orthopedic Foot and Ankle Society® (AOFAS) for 9 years from 2013 until 2022. Dr. Doug spends part of his professional time optimizing patients on his two platforms. The remainder of his time is spent spearheading a worldwide campaign to educate patients on the facts around hormone replacement and osteoporosis through virtual and in-person talks as well as creation of digital content for YouTube and The Dr. Doug Show podcast.

In his personal time, Dr. Doug recharges by connecting with his phenomenal wife, Dr. Ashley Lucas, and their three children. He is an avid outdoor enthusiast and enjoys hiking, cycling, surfing and snow sports. His deep passion for health permeates every aspect of his life and is easily reflected in those in contact with him.

RESOURCES

YouTube:

https://www.youtube.com/@Dr_DougLucas

https://www.youtube.com/@PEMABioIdentical

Facebook:

https://www.facebook.com/DrDougLucas

https://www.facebook.com/PEMABioIdentical

Instagram:

https://www.instagram.com/dr_douglucas

https://www.instagram.com/PEMABioIdentical

Podcast:

Listen on Spotify & Apple Podcasts

Website:

https://PEMABioIdentical.com

REFERENCES

REASON #2–NOT USING ESTROGEN DUE TO FEAR OF BREAST CANCER AND BLOOD CLOTS

1. Glaser RL, York AE, Dimitrakakis C. Incidence of invasive breast cancer in women treated with testosterone implants: a prospective 10-year cohort study. BMC Cancer. 2019 Dec 30;19 (1):1271. doi: 10.1186/s12885-019-6457-8. PMID: 31888528; PMCID: PMC6937705.

2. Hofling M, Hirschberg AL, Skoog L, Tani E, Hägerström T, von Schoultz B. Testosterone inhibits estrogen/progestogen-induced breast cell proliferation in postmenopausal women. Menopause. 2007 Mar-Apr;14(2):183-90. doi: 10.1097/01.gme.0000232033.92411.51. PMID: 17108847.

3. Dimitrakakis C, Bondy C. Androgens and the breast. Breast Cancer Res. 2009;11(5):212. doi: 10.1186/bcr2413. PMID: 19889198; PMCID: PMC2790857.

4. van Staa TP, Sprafka JM. Study of adverse outcomes in women using testosterone therapy. Maturitas. 2009 Jan 20;62(1):76-80. doi: 10.1016/j.maturitas.2008.11.001. Epub 2008 Dec 24. PMID: 19108962.

5. Islam RM, Bell RJ, Green S, Page MJ, Davis SR. Safety and efficacy of testosterone for women: a systematic review and meta-analysis of randomised controlled trial data. Lancet Diabetes Endocrinol. 2019 Oct;7(10):754-766. doi: 10.1016/S2213-8587(19)30189-5. Epub 2019 Jul 25. PMID: 31353194.

6. Zang H, Carlström K, Arner P, Hirschberg AL. Effects of treatment with testosterone alone or in combination with estrogen on insulin sensitivity in postmenopausal women. Fertil Steril. 2006 Jul;86(1):136-44. doi: 10.1016/j.fertnstert.2005.12.039. Epub 2006 Jun 5. PMID: 16750207.

7. Rossouw JE, Anderson GL, Prentice RL, LaCroix AZ, Kooperberg C, Stefanick ML, Jackson RD, Beresford SA, Howard BV, Johnson KC, Kotchen JM, Ockene J; Writing Group for the Women's Health Initiative Investigators. Risks and benefits of estrogen plus progestin in healthy postmenopausal women: principal results From the Women's Health Initiative randomized controlled trial. JAMA. 2002 Jul 17;288(3):321-33. doi: 10.1001/jama.288.3.321. PMID: 12117397.

8. Anderson GL, Limacher M, Assaf AR, Bassford T, Beresford SA, Black H, Bonds D, Brunner R, Brzyski R, Caan B, Chlebowski R, Curb D, Gass M, Hays J, Heiss G, Hendrix S, Howard BV, Hsia J, Hubbell A, Jackson R, Johnson KC, Judd H, Kotchen JM, Kuller L, LaCroix AZ, Lane D, Langer RD, Lasser N, Lewis CE, Manson J, Margolis K, Ockene J, O'Sullivan MJ, Phillips L, Prentice RL, Ritenbaugh C, Robbins J, Rossouw JE, Sarto G, Stefanick ML, Van Horn L, Wactawski-Wende J, Wallace R, Wassertheil-Smoller S; Women's Health Initiative Steering Committee. Effects of conjugated equine estrogen in postmenopausal women with hysterectomy: the Women's Health Initiative randomized controlled trial. JAMA. 2004 Apr 14;291 (14):1701-12. doi: 10.1001/jama.291.14.1701. PMID: 15082697.

9. Manson JE, Crandall CJ, Rossouw JE, Chlebowski RT, Anderson GL, Stefanick ML, Aragaki AK, Cauley JA, Wells GL, LaCroix AZ, Thomson CA, Neuhouser ML, Van Horn L, Kooperberg C, Howard BV, Tinker LF, Wactawski-Wende J, Shumaker SA, Prentice RL. The Women's Health Initiative Randomized Trials and Clinical Practice: A Review. JAMA. 2024 May 1. doi: 10.1001/jama.2024.6542. Epub ahead of print. PMID: 38691368.

10. Lalitkumar PGL, Lundström E, Byström B, Ujvari D, Murkes D, Tani E, Söderqvist G. Effects of Estradiol/Micronized Progesterone vs. Conjugated Equine Estrogens/Medroxyprogesterone Acetate on Breast Cancer Gene Expression in Healthy Postmenopausal Women. Int J Mol Sci. 2023 Feb 18;24(4):4123. doi: 10.3390/ijms24044123. PMID: 36835533; PMCID: PMC9959219.

11. Simin J, Tamimi R, Lagergren J, Adami HO, Brusselaers N. Menopausal hormone therapy and cancer risk: An overestimated risk? Eur J Cancer. 2017 Oct;84:60-68. doi: 10.1016/j.ejca.2017.07.012. Epub 2017 Aug 4. PMID: 28783542.

12. Abenhaim HA, Suissa S, Azoulay L, Spence AR, Czuzoj-Shulman N, Tulandi T. Menopausal Hormone Therapy Formulation and Breast Cancer Risk. Obstet Gynecol. 2022 Jun 1;139(6):1103-1110. doi: 10.1097/AOG.0000000000004723. Epub 2022 May 3. PMID: 35675607.

13. Beral V; Million Women Study Collaborators. Breast cancer and hormone-replacement therapy in the Million Women Study. Lancet. 2003 Aug 9;362(9382):419-27. doi: 10.1016/s0140-6736(03)14065-2. Erratum in: Lancet. 2003 Oct 4;362(9390):1160. PMID: 12927427.

14. Graham S, Archer DF, Simon JA, Ohleth KM, Bernick B. Review of menopausal hormone therapy with estradiol and progesterone versus other estrogens and progestins. Gynecol Endocrinol. 2022 Nov;38(11):891-910. doi: 10.1080/09513590.2022.2118254. Epub 2022 Sep 8. PMID: 36075250.

15. Mikkola TS, Savolainen-Peltonen H, Tuomikoski P, Hoti F, Vattulainen P, Gissler M, Ylikorkala O. Reduced risk of breast cancer mortality in women using postmenopausal hormone therapy: a Finnish nationwide comparative study. Menopause. 2016 Nov;23(11):1199-1203. doi: 10.1097/GME.0000000000000698. PMID: 27465718.

16. Shapiro S, Farmer RD, Stevenson JC, Burger HG, Mueck AO. Does hormone replacement therapy cause breast cancer? An application of causal principles to three studies. Part 4: the Million Women Study. J Fam Plann Reprod Health Care. 2012 Apr;38(2):102-9. doi: 10.1136/jfprhc-2011-100229. Epub 2012 Jan 16. PMID: 22262621.

17. Roach RE, Helmerhorst FM, Lijfering WM, Stijnen T, Algra A, Dekkers OM. Combined oral contraceptives: the risk of myocardial infarction and ischemic stroke. Cochrane Database Syst Rev. 2015 Aug 27;2015(8):CD011054. doi: 10.1002/14651858.CD011054.pub2. PMID: 26310586; PMCID: PMC6494192.

18. Panay N, Nappi RE, Stute P, Palacios S, Paszkowski T, Kagan R, Archer DF, Héroux J, Boolell M. Oral estradiol/micronized progesterone may be associated with lower risk of venous thromboembolism compared with conjugated equine estrogens/medroxyprogesterone acetate in real-world practice. Maturitas. 2023 Jun;172:23-31. doi: 10.1016/j.maturitas.2023.04.004. Epub 2023 Apr 13. PMID: 37084589.

19. Vinogradova Y, Coupland C, Hippisley-Cox J. Use of hormone replacement therapy and risk of venous thromboembolism: nested case-control studies using the QResearch and CPRD databases. BMJ. 2019 Jan 9;364:k4810. doi: 10.1136/bmj.k4810. Erratum in: BMJ. 2019 Jan 15;364:l162. PMID: 30626577; PMCID: PMC6326068.

REASON #3–NOT USING PROGESTERONE BECAUSE YOU DON'T HAVE A UTERUS

1. Chaudhry A, Puntis ML, Gikas P, Mokbel K. Does the timing of breast cancer surgery in premenopausal women affect clinical outcome? An update. Int Semin Surg Oncol. 2006 Nov 1;3:37. doi: 10.1186/1477-7800-3-37. PMID: 17078874; PMCID: PMC1635554.

2. Prior JC. Progesterone for the prevention and treatment of osteoporosis in women. Climacteric. 2018 Aug;21(4):366-374. doi: 10.1080/13697137.2018.1467400. Epub 2018 Jul 2. PMID: 29962257.

3. Rossouw JE, Anderson GL, Prentice RL, LaCroix AZ, Kooperberg C, Stefanick ML, Jackson RD, Beresford SA, Howard BV, Johnson KC, Kotchen JM, Ockene J; Writing Group for the Women's Health Initiative Investigators. Risks and benefits of estrogen plus progestin in healthy postmenopausal women: principal results From the Women's Health Initiative randomized controlled trial. JAMA. 2002 Jul 17;288(3):321-33. doi: 10.1001/jama.288.3.321. PMID: 12117397.

4. Formby B, Wiley TS. Progesterone inhibits growth and induces apoptosis in breast cancer cells: inverse effects on Bcl-2 and p53. Ann Clin Lab Sci. 1998 Nov-Dec;28(6):360-9. PMID: 9846203.

5. Løkkegaard E, Andreasen AH, Jacobsen RK, Nielsen LH, Agger C, Lidegaard Ø. Hormone therapy and risk of myocardial infarction: a national register study. Eur Heart J. 2008 Nov;29(21):2660-8. doi: 10.1093/eurheartj/ehn408. Epub 2008 Sep 30. PMID: 18826989.

6. Hitchcock CL, Prior JC. Oral micronized progesterone for vasomotor symptoms--a placebo-controlled randomized trial in healthy postmenopausal women. Menopause. 2012 Aug;19(8):886-93. doi: 10.1097/gme.0b013e318247f07a. PMID: 22453200.

7. dos Santos RL, da Silva FB, Ribeiro RF Jr, Stefanon I. Sex hormones in the cardiovascular system. Horm Mol Biol Clin Investig. 2014 May;18(2):89-103. doi: 10.1515/hmbci-2013-0048. PMID: 25390005.

8. Baik SH, Baye F, McDonald CJ. Use of menopausal hormone therapy beyond age 65 years and its effects on women's health outcomes by types, routes, and doses. Menopause. 2024 May 1;31(5):363-371. doi: 10.1097/GME.0000000000002335. Epub 2024 Mar 9. PMID: 38595196.

9. Schumacher M, Sitruk-Ware R, De Nicola AF. Progesterone and progestins: neuroprotection and myelin repair. Curr Opin Pharmacol. 2008 Dec;8(6):740-6. doi: 10.1016/j.coph.2008.10.002. Epub 2008 Nov 6. Erratum in: Curr Opin Pharmacol. 2009 Apr;9(2):227. PMID: 18929681.

REASON #4–IGNORING STRESS AND ADRENAL HEALTH

1. Travison, T., Araujo, A., O'Donnell, A., Kupelian, V., & McKinlay, J. (2007). A Population-Level Decline in Serum Testosterone Levels in American Men. Journal of Clinical Endocrinology and Metabolism, 92(1), 196-202.

2. Zumoff B, Strain GW, Miller LK, Rosner W. Twenty-four-hour mean plasma testosterone concentration declines with age in normal premenopausal women. J Clin Endocrinol Metab. 1995 Apr;80(4):1429-30. doi: 10.1210/jcem.80.4.7714119. PMID: 7714119.

REASON #5–IGNORING TESTOSTERONE

1. Glaser R, Dimitrakakis C. Testosterone therapy in women: myths and misconceptions. Maturitas. 2013 Mar;74(3):230-4. doi: 10.1016/j.maturitas.2013.01.003. Epub 2013 Feb 4. PMID: 23380529.

2. Davis SR, Baber R, Panay N, Bitzer J, Perez SC, Islam RM, Kaunitz AM, Kingsberg SA, Lambrinoudaki I, Liu J, Parish SJ, Pinkerton J, Rymer J, Simon JA, Vignozzi L, Wierman ME. Global Consensus Position Statement on the Use of Testosterone Therapy for Women. J Clin Endocrinol Metab. 2019 Oct 1;104(10):4660-4666. doi: 10.1210/jc.2019-01603. PMID: 31498871; PMCID: PMC6821450.

3. Wierman ME, Basson R, Davis SR, Khosla S, Miller KK, Rosner W, Santoro N. Androgen therapy in women: an Endocrine Society Clinical Practice guideline. J Clin Endocrinol Metab. 2006 Oct;91(10):3697-710. doi: 10.1210/jc.2006-1121. Epub 2006 Oct 3. Erratum in: J Clin Endocrinol Metab. 2021 Jun 16;106(7):e2850. PMID: 17018650.

4. Glaser R, York AE, Dimitrakakis C. Beneficial effects of testosterone therapy in women measured by the validated Menopause Rating Scale (MRS). Maturitas. 2011 Apr;68(4):355-61. doi: 10.1016/j.maturitas.2010.12.001. Epub 2010 Dec 21. PMID: 21177051.

5. Glaser R, Dimitrakakis C. Testosterone therapy in women: myths and misconceptions. Maturitas. 2013 Mar;74(3):230-4. doi: 10.1016/j.maturitas.2013.01.003. Epub 2013 Feb 4. PMID: 23380529.

6. Glaser R, York AE, Dimitrakakis C. Beneficial effects of testosterone therapy in women measured by the validated Menopause Rating Scale (MRS). Maturitas. 2011 Apr;68(4):355-61. doi: 10.1016/j.maturitas.2010.12.001. Epub 2010 Dec 21. PMID: 21177051.

7. Goldstat R, Briganti E, Tran J, Wolfe R, Davis SR. Transdermal testosterone therapy improves well-being, mood, and sexual function in premenopausal women. Menopause. 2003 Sep-Oct;10(5):390-8. doi: 10.1097/01.GME.0000060256.03945.20. PMID: 14501599.

8. Miller KK, Grieco KA, Klibanski A. Testosterone administration in women with anorexia nervosa. J Clin Endocrinol Metab. 2005 Mar;90(3):1428-33. doi: 10.1210/jc.2004-1181. Epub 2004 Dec 21. PMID: 15613421.

9. Britto R, Araújo L, Barbosa I, Silva L, Rocha S, Valente AP. Hormonal therapy with estradiol and testosterone implants: bone protection? Gynecol Endocrinol. 2011 Feb;27(2):96-100. doi: 10.3109/09513590.2010.489131. Epub 2010 May 26. PMID: 20504104.

10. Davis SR, McCloud P, Strauss BJ, Burger H. Testosterone enhances estradiol's effects on postmenopausal bone density and sexuality. Maturitas. 2008 Sep-Oct;61(1-2):17-26. doi: 10.1016/j.maturitas.2008.09.006. PMID: 19434876.

11. Buratto J, Kirk B, Phu S, Vogrin S, Duque G. Safety and Efficacy of Testosterone Therapy on Musculoskeletal Health and Clinical Outcomes in Men: A Systematic Review and Meta-Analysis of Randomized Placebo-Controlled Trials. Endocr Pract. 2023 Sep;29(9):727-734. doi: 10.1016/j.eprac.2023.04.013. Epub 2023 May 8. PMID: 37164187.

12. Shifren JL, Davis SR, Moreau M, Waldbaum A, Bouchard C, DeRogatis L, Derzko C, Bearnson P, Kakos N, O'Neill S, Levine S, Wekselman K, Buch A, Rodenberg C, Kroll R. Testosterone patch for the treatment of hypoactive sexual desire disorder in naturally menopausal women: results from the INTIMATE NM1 Study. Menopause. 2006 Sep-Oct;13(5):770-9. doi: 10.1097/01.gme.0000243567.32828.99. Erratum in: Menopause. 2007 Jan-Feb;14(1):157. PMID: 16932240.

13. Davis SR, van der Mooren MJ, van Lunsen RH, Lopes P, Ribot C, Rees M, Moufarege A, Rodenberg C, Buch A, Purdie DW. Efficacy and safety of a testosterone patch for the treatment of hypoactive sexual desire disorder in surgically menopausal women: a randomized, placebo-controlled trial. Menopause. 2006 May-Jun;13(3):387-96. doi:

10.1097/01.gme.0000179049.08371.c7. Erratum in: Menopause. 2006 Sep-Oct;13(5):850. Ribot, Jean [corrected to Ribot, Claude]. PMID: 16735935.

14. Braunstein GD, Sundwall DA, Katz M, Shifren JL, Buster JE, Simon JA, Bachman G, Aguirre OA, Lucas JD, Rodenberg C, Buch A, Watts NB. Safety and efficacy of a testosterone patch for the treatment of hypoactive sexual desire disorder in surgically menopausal women: a randomized, placebo-controlled trial. Arch Intern Med. 2005 Jul 25;165(14):1582-9. doi: 10.1001/archinte.165.14.1582. PMID: 16043675.

15. Alkatib AA, Cosma M, Elamin MB, Erickson D, Swiglo BA, Erwin PJ, Montori VM. A systematic review and meta-analysis of randomized placebo-controlled trials of DHEA treatment effects on quality of life in women with adrenal insufficiency. J Clin Endocrinol Metab. 2009 Oct;94(10):3676-81. doi: 10.1210/jc.2009-0672. Epub 2009 Sep 22. PMID: 19773400.

16. Guo W, Bachman E, Li M, Roy CN, Blusztajn J, Wong S, Chan SY, Serra C, Jasuja R, Travison TG, Muckenthaler MU, Nemeth E, Bhasin S. Testosterone administration inhibits hepcidin transcription and is associated with increased iron incor-

poration into red blood cells. Aging Cell. 2013 Apr;12(2):280-91. doi: 10.1111/acel.12052. Epub 2013 Feb 28. PMID: 23399021; PMCID: PMC3602280.

17. Gabrielsen, J.S. Iron and Testosterone: Interplay and Clinical Implications. Curr Sex Health Rep 9, 5–11 (2017). https://doi.org/10.1007/s11930-017-0097-2

REASON #6–YOU'RE "TOO OLD" TO START HRT OR "TOO OLD" TO CONTINUE HRT (HEART AND BRAIN HEALTH)

1. Naftolin F, Friedenthal J, Nachtigall R, Nachtigall L. Cardiovascular health and the menopausal woman: the role of estrogen and when to begin and end hormone treatment. F1000Res. 2019 Sep 3;8:F1000 Faculty Rev-1576. doi: 10.12688/f1000research.15548.1. PMID: 31543950; PMCID: PMC6733383.

2. Chester RC, Kling JM, Manson JE. What the Women's Health Initiative has taught us about menopausal hormone therapy. Clin Cardiol. 2018 Feb;41(2):247-252. doi: 10.1002/clc.22891. Epub 2018 Mar 1. PMID: 29493798; PMCID: PMC6490107.

3. Harman SM, Black DM, Naftolin F, Brinton EA, Budoff MJ, Cedars MI, Hopkins PN, Lobo RA, Manson JE, Merriam GR, Miller VM, Neal-Perry G, Santoro N, Taylor HS, Vittinghoff E, Yan M, Hodis HN. Arterial imaging outcomes and cardiovascular risk factors in recently menopausal women: a randomized trial. Ann Intern Med. 2014 Aug 19;161(4):249-60. doi: 10.7326/M14-0353. PMID: 25069991.

4. Bhupathiraju SN, Grodstein F, Rosner BA, Stampfer MJ, Hu FB, Willett WC, Manson JE. Hormone Therapy Use and Risk of Chronic Disease in the Nurses' Health Study: A Comparative Analysis With the Women's Health Initiative. Am J Epidemiol. 2017 Sep 15;186(6):696-708. doi: 10.1093/aje/kwx131. Erratum in: Am J Epidemiol. 2018 Mar 1;187(3):636. PMID: 28938710; PMCID: PMC5860527.

5. Schierbeck LL, Rejnmark L, Tofteng CL, Stilgren L, Eiken P, Mosekilde L, Køber L, Jensen JE. Effect of hormone replacement therapy on cardiovascular events in recently postmenopausal women: randomised trial. BMJ. 2012 Oct 9;345:e6409. doi: 10.1136/bmj.e6409. PMID: 23048011.

6. Bhupathiraju SN, Grodstein F, Stampfer MJ, Willett WC, Hu FB, Manson JE. Exogenous Hormone Use: Oral Contraceptives, Postmenopausal Hormone Therapy, and Health Outcomes in the Nurses' Health Study. Am J Public Health. 2016 Sep;106(9):1631-7. doi: 10.2105/AJPH.2016.303349. Epub 2016 Jul 26. PMID: 27459451; PMCID: PMC4981817.

7. Manson JE, Aragaki AK, Rossouw JE, Anderson GL, Prentice RL, LaCroix AZ, Chlebowski RT, Howard BV, Thomson CA, Margolis KL, Lewis CE, Stefanick ML, Jackson RD, Johnson KC, Martin LW, Shumaker SA, Espeland MA, Wactawski-Wende J; WHI Investigators. Menopausal Hormone Therapy and Long-term All-Cause and Cause-Specific Mortality: The Women's Health Initiative Randomized Trials. JAMA. 2017 Sep 12;318(10):927-938. doi: 10.1001/jama.2017.11217. PMID: 28898378; PMCID: PMC5728370.

8. Dimitrakakis C, Bondy C. Androgens and the breast. Breast Cancer Res. 2009;11(5):212. doi: 10.1186/bcr2413. PMID: 19889198; PMCID: PMC2790857.

9. Nerattini M, Jett S, Andy C, Carlton C, Zarate C, Boneu C, Battista M, Pahlajani S, Loeb-Zeitlin S, Havryulik Y, Williams S, Christos P, Fink M, Brinton RD, Mosconi L. Systematic review and meta-analysis of the effects of menopause hormone therapy on risk of Alzheimer's disease and dementia. Front Aging Neurosci. 2023 Oct 23;15:1260427. doi: 10.3389/fnagi.2023.1260427. PMID: 37937120; PMCID: PMC10625913.

10. Baik SH, Baye F, McDonald CJ. Use of menopausal hormone therapy beyond age 65 years and its effects on women's health outcomes by types, routes, and doses. Menopause. 2024 May 1;31(5):363-371. doi: 10.1097/GME.0000000000002335. Epub 2024 Mar 9. PMID: 38595196.

REASON #7–MAYBE YOU SIMPLY NEED MORE?

1. Lo JC, Burnett-Bowie SA, Finkelstein JS. Bone and the perimenopause. Obstet Gynecol Clin North Am. 2011 Sep;38(3):503-17. doi: 10.1016/j.ogc.2011.07.001. PMID: 21961717; PMCID: PMC3920744.

2. Reginster JY, Sarlet N, Deroisy R, Albert A, Gaspard U, Franchimont P. Minimal levels of serum estradiol prevent postmenopausal bone loss. Calcif Tissue Int. 1992 Nov;51(5):340-3. doi: 10.1007/BF00316876. PMID: 1458336.

3. Zhu Z, Zhao J, Fang Y, Hua R. Association between serum estradiol level, sex hormone binding globulin level, and bone mineral density in middle-aged postmenopausal women. J Orthop Surg Res. 2021 Oct 30;16(1):648. doi: 10.1186/s13018-021-02799-3. PMID: 34717706; PMCID: PMC8557509.

4. Huitrón-Bravo G, Denova-Gutiérrez E, Talavera JO, Moran-Villota C, Tamayo J, Omaña-Covarrubias A, Salmerón J. Levels of serum estradiol and lifestyle factors related with bone mineral density in premenopausal Mexican women: a cross-sectional analysis. BMC Musculoskelet Disord. 2016 Oct 19;17(1):437. doi: 10.1186/s12891-016-1273-7. PMID: 27756278; PMCID: PMC5069822.

5. Zhu Z, Zhao J, Fang Y, Hua R. Association between serum estradiol level, sex hormone binding globulin level, and bone mineral density in middle-aged postmenopausal women. J Orthop Surg Res. 2021 Oct 30;16(1):648. doi: 10.1186/s13018-021-02799-3. PMID: 34717706; PMCID: PMC8557509.

6. Hadji P, Colli E, Regidor PA. Bone health in estrogen-free contraception. Osteoporos Int. 2019 Dec;30(12):2391-2400. doi: 10.1007/s00198-019-05103-6. Epub 2019 Aug 24. Erratum in: Osteoporos Int. 2020 Jul;31(7):1399. PMID: 31446440; PMCID: PMC7203087.

7. Reginster JY, Sarlet N, Deroisy R, Albert A, Gaspard U, Franchimont P. Minimal levels of serum estradiol prevent postmenopausal bone loss. Calcif Tissue Int. 1992 Nov;51(5):340-3. doi: 10.1007/BF00316876. PMID: 1458336.

8. Yang TS, Chen YJ, Liang WH, Chang CY, Tai LC, Chang SP, Ng HT. A clinical trial of 3 doses of transdermal 17beta-estradiol for preventing postmenopausal bone loss: a preliminary study. J Chin Med Assoc. 2007 May;70(5):200-6. doi: 10.1016/S1726-4901(09)70358-2. PMID: 17524997.

9. Stanosz S, Zochowska E, Safranow K, Sieja K, Stanosz M. Influence of modified transdermal hormone replacement therapy on the concentrations of hormones, growth factors, and bone mineral density in women with osteopenia. Metabolism. 2009 Jan;58(1):1-7. doi: 10.1016/j.metabol.2008.07.016. PMID: 19059524.

REASON #8–MAYBE YOU NEED TO MENSTRUATE?

1. Løkkegaard E, Andreasen AH, Jacobsen RK, Nielsen LH, Agger C, Lidegaard Ø. Hormone therapy and risk of myocardial infarction: a national register study. Eur Heart J. 2008 Nov;29 (21):2660-8. doi: 10.1093/eurheartj/ehn408. Epub 2008 Sep 30. PMID: 18826989.

2. Gonnelli S, Cepollaro C, Pondrelli C, Martini S, Monaco R, Gennari C. The usefulness of bone turnover in predicting the response to transdermal estrogen therapy in postmenopausal osteoporosis. J Bone Miner Res. 1997 Apr;12(4):624-31. doi: 10.1359/jbmr.1997.12.4.624. PMID: 9101374.

3. Adami S, Suppi R, Bertoldo F, Rossini M, Residori M, Maresca V, Lo Cascio V. Transdermal estradiol in the treatment of postmenopausal bone loss. Bone Miner. 1989 Aug;7(1):79-86. doi: 10.1016/0169-6009(89)90064-0. PMID: 2670019.

4. Yang TS, Chen YJ, Liang WH, Chang CY, Tai LC, Chang SP, Ng HT. A clinical trial of 3 doses of transdermal 17beta-estradiol for preventing postmenopausal bone loss: a preliminary study. J Chin Med Assoc. 2007 May;70(5):200-6. doi:

10.1016/S1726-4901(09)70358-2. PMID: 17524997.

5. Stanosz S, Zochowska E, Safranow K, Sieja K, Stanosz M. Influence of modified transdermal hormone replacement therapy on the concentrations of hormones, growth factors, and bone mineral density in women with osteopenia. Metabolism. 2009 Jan;58(1):1-7. doi: 10.1016/j.metabol.2008.07.016. PMID: 19059524.

6. Hosking D, Chilvers CE, Christiansen C, Ravn P, Wasnich R, Ross P, McClung M, Balske A, Thompson D, Daley M, Yates AJ. Prevention of bone loss with alendronate in postmenopausal women under 60 years of age. Early Postmenopausal Intervention Cohort Study Group. N Engl J Med. 1998 Feb 19;338(8):485-92. doi: 10.1056/NEJM199802193380801. PMID: 9443925.

7. Ettinger B, Ensrud KE, Wallace R, Johnson KC, Cummings SR, Yankov V, Vittinghoff E, Grady D. Effects of ultralow-dose transdermal estradiol on bone mineral density: a randomized clinical trial. Obstet Gynecol. 2004 Sep;104(3):443-51. doi: 10.1097/01.AOG.0000137833.43248.79. PMID: 15339752.

8. Seifert-Klauss V, Prior JC. Progesterone and bone: actions promoting bone health in women. J Osteoporos. 2010 Oct 31;2010:845180. doi: 10.4061/2010/845180. PMID: 21052538; PMCID: PMC2968416.

9. Ramakrishnan R, Khan SA, Badve S. Morphological changes in breast tissue with menstrual cycle. Mod Pathol. 2002 Dec;15(12):1348-56. doi: 10.1097/01.MP.0000039566.20817.46. PMID: 12481017.

10. Formby B, Wiley TS. Progesterone inhibits growth and induces apoptosis in breast cancer cells: inverse effects on Bcl-2 and p53. Ann Clin Lab Sci. 1998 Nov-Dec;28(6):360-9. PMID: 9846203.

11. Azeez JM, Sithul H, Hariharan I, Sreekumar S, Prabhakar J, Sreeja S, Pillai MR. Progesterone regulates the proliferation of breast cancer cells - in vitro evidence. Drug Des Devel Ther. 2015 Nov 9;9:5987-99. doi: 10.2147/DDDT.S89390. PMID: 26609221; PMCID: PMC4644174.

12. Cowan LD, Gordis L, Tonascia JA, Jones GS. Breast cancer incidence in women with a history of progesterone deficiency. Am J Epidemiol. 1981 Aug;114(2):209-17. doi: 10.1093/oxfordjournals.aje.a113184. PMID: 7304556.

13. Jatoi I. Timing of surgery for primary breast cancer with regard to the menstrual phase and prognosis. Breast Cancer Res Treat. 1998;52(1-3):217-25. doi: 10.1023/a:1006121117336. PMID: 10066084.

14. Fadini GP, de Kreutzenberg S, Albiero M, Coracina A, Pagnin E, Baesso I, Cignarella A, Bolego C, Plebani M, Nardelli GB, Sartore S, Agostini C, Avogaro A. Gender differences in endothelial progenitor cells and cardiovascular risk profile: the role of female estrogens. Arterioscler Thromb Vasc Biol. 2008 May;28(5):997-1004. doi: 10.1161/ATVBAHA.107.159558. Epub 2008 Feb 14. PMID: 18276910.

15. Hosking D, Chilvers CE, Christiansen C, Ravn P, Wasnich R, Ross P, McClung M, Balske A, Thompson D, Daley M, Yates AJ. Prevention of bone loss with alendronate in postmenopausal women under 60 years of age. Early Postmenopausal Intervention Cohort Study Group. N Engl J Med. 1998 Feb 19;338(8):485-92. doi: 10.1056/NEJM199802193380801. PMID: 9443925.

REASON #9–YOU'RE STRUGGLING TO PUT IT ALL TOGETHER!

1. Reginster JY, Sarlet N, Deroisy R, Albert A, Gaspard U, Franchimont P. Minimal levels of serum estradiol prevent postmenopausal bone loss. Calcif Tissue Int. 1992 Nov;51(5):340-3. doi: 10.1007/BF00316876. PMID: 1458336.

2. Yang TS, Chen YJ, Liang WH, Chang CY, Tai LC, Chang SP, Ng HT. A clinical trial of 3 doses of transdermal 17beta-estradiol for preventing postmenopausal bone loss: a preliminary study. J Chin Med Assoc. 2007 May;70(5):200-6. doi: 10.1016/S1726-4901(09)70358-2. PMID: 17524997.

3. Dimitrakakis C, Bondy C. Androgens and the breast. Breast Cancer Res. 2009;11(5):212. doi: 10.1186/bcr2413. PMID: 19889198; PMCID: PMC2790857.

THANK YOU!

Thank you for reading this short book on hormone optimization for women. As a special thank you for spending your precious time with me, I'd like to offer you a some free gifts.

Please head over to:

https://PEMABioIdentical.com/book

for additional resources and materials to help you on your journey.

www.ingramcontent.com/pod-product-compliance
Lightning Source LLC
Chambersburg PA
CBHW052253220526
45471CB00001B/324